THE SUPERVISORY RELATIONSHIP

The Supervisory Relationship

A Contemporary Psychodynamic Approach

Mary Gail Frawley-O'Dea, PhD
Joan E. Sarnat, PhD

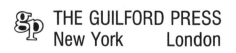 THE GUILFORD PRESS
New York   London

© 2001 The Guilford Press
A Division of Guilford Publications, Inc.
72 Spring Street, New York, NY 10012
www.guilford.com

Printed in the United States of America

This book is printed on acid-free paper.

Last digit is print number: 9   8   7   6   5   4   3   2

Library of Congress Cataloging-in-Publication Data

Frawley-O'Dea, Mary Gail, 1950–
    The supervisory relationship : a contemporary psychodynamic approach /
    Mary Gail Frawley-O'Dea, Joan E. Sarnat.
       p.   cm.
    Includes bibliographical references and index.
    ISBN 1-57230-621-1
      1. Psychoanalysis—Study and teaching—Supervision. 2. Psychodynamic
    psychotherapy—Study and teaching—Supervision. 3. Psychotherapists—
    Supervision of.   I. Sarnat, Joan E.   II. Title.

RC502.F73 2001
616.89′14—dc21   00-061697

Chapter 6 is based on Sarnat (1998). Chapter 7 is based on Frawley-O'Dea
(1998). Both copyright 1998 by The American Academy of Psychoanalysis.
Adapted by permission.

For my beloved O'Deas: my husband, Dennis;
my daughter, Mollie; my stepson, Daniel; my Bosnian
stepson, Igor Ibradzic "O'Dea"; and to the memory
of my stepmother-in-law, Johanna
—M. G. F.-O.

For David, Jascha, and Michael
—J. E. S.

About the Authors

Mary Gail Frawley-O'Dea, PhD, is a faculty member and supervisor at the Derner Institute for Advanced Psychological Studies at Adelphi University, Garden City, New York; the Minnesota Institute for Contemporary Psychoanalytic Studies; and the National Training Program in Contemporary Psychoanalysis in New York City. She also is on the continuing education faculty of the National Psychological Association for Psychoanalysis, Inc., in New York City. Coauthor with Jody Messler Davies of *Treating the Adult Survivor of Childhood Sexual Abuse: A Psychoanalytic Perspective,* Dr. Frawley-O'Dea is a clinical psychologist and psychoanalyst in clinical and supervisory practice in New City, New York.

Joan E. Sarnat, PhD, is a clinical psychologist in private practice in Berkeley, California. She is Board Certified in Clinical Psychology by the American Board of Professional Psychology and is a member of the Psychoanalytic Institute of Northern California. She is on the adjunct faculties of the California School of Professional Psychology and The Wright Institute, Berkeley, California. She has supervised and led case conferences for over 20 years, and conducts consultation groups for supervisors.

Acknowledgments

Mary Gail Frawley-O'Dea

When Joan and I met with Kitty Moore at The Guilford Press to discuss with her our ideas for a book on supervision, we barely knew each other. Four years later, this situation has changed dramatically. During the process of cowriting this book with Joan, I have come to know her well, and I am filled with gratitude for her participation in this project. Over the past 4 years, I have learned to appreciate and rely on Joan's intellectual prowess, theoretical facility, clinical acuity, and fine writing. In addition, her intellectual integrity—her insistence and persistence in ensuring that the book reach and sustain a standard of clarity, completeness, and complexity—greatly enriched the process of coauthorship for me. Beyond these professional qualities, I value deeply Joan's friendship and sense of humor. We played, we argued, and we supported each other personally and professionally. We are colleagues and we are friends, and I have grown through both of those relationships with Joan. Thank you, Joan.

This book's gestation began for me during my supervision with Irwin Hirsch. Irwin and I have written elsewhere of our supervisory year together (Frawley-O'Dea, 1997a; Hirsch, 1997). Although our supervisory relationship was disappointing to both of us at the time, our subsequent processing of that experience led not only to the seedbed for this book but also to a collegial and personal relationship with Irwin that is meaningful to me. His rigorous intellectual and personal integrity, his warmth, humor, and, most important, his profound generativity have contributed directly to this project. He generously read the initial manuscript of this book, and his comments significantly enhanced the finished product. My thanks to Irwin for his professional support and for his friendship.

Jonathan Slavin also has been a friend and advisor for almost a decade. At a time of change and challenge in his own life, Jonathan read the first draft of this book and offered suggestions that helped us improve a number of sections of the final manuscript. I am grateful to him for all his personal and professional support over the years.

Sandra Buechler, who herself has written about the supervisory relationship, was kind enough to read a portion of the manuscript and made a number of pertinent editorial suggestions. I thank her for giving the project some time when she had little of it to spare. I also thank Charles Spezzano and Sue Elkind, who reviewed the manuscript and offered thoughtful comments and suggestions.

Both my doctoral and postdoctoral training took place at the Derner Institute for Advanced Psychological Studies at Adelphi University. From my first year of doctoral training through my last year of post-doc, I was fortunate to work with supervisors who challenged me intellectually and clinically, while supporting me as a developing clinician/analyst and as a person with unique strengths, deficits, and ways of working. Each supervisor lives on in the analytic voice I developed during my training and, thus, in the ideas presented in this book. I am thankful to the "Baldwin band": Doug Milman, Fred Woolverton, Sheri Fenster, and Elyse Billow, and to Jerry Gold, Marty Fisher, Michael Zentman, Bob Mendelsohn, Irwin Hirsch, Joe Newirth, and Muriel Dimen for all that I learned from them. Numerous gifted analysts facilitated case conferences in both my doctoral and postdoctoral programs, and I learned much from them and my colleagues during those clinical discussions. I would like to mention especially the late Bruce Kopp, whose conceptualization of unconscious fantasy helped me finally understand this concept in a clinically useful way. His untimely death deprived the Derner postdoctoral program of a decent man and a generous teacher.

I thank George Stricker, Bob Mendelsohn, Jonathan Jackson, and Joe Newirth for encouraging my more recent development as a faculty member and supervisor at Derner. There and in my private practice, I have been privileged to work with supervisees whose intelligence, clinical talent, dedication, and willingness to reflect on themselves, the clinical relationship in which they are involved, and their supervisory relationship with me have enhanced my own continued personal and professional growth. Their direct and indirect contributions to my thinking are detectable in these pages.

Kitty Moore believed in this project and gave us the chance to write the book, with the security that we had a publisher supporting our work. Jim Nageotte then took over this project. I have appreciated Jim's responsiveness, sense of humor, and editorial vision. He has made the business end of this project easy.

Writing a book, even with a coauthor as available and engaged as Joan, is a long, often frustrating, always time-consuming process. For 4 years, the book was always somewhere on my mind, and especially for the last year, I was often immersed in writing and therefore unavailable to friends and family. My friends' support and understanding have sustained me, and I am appreciative of their constancy. Judy Weiss-Brown and Howie Brown, Richard and Jane Gartner, David Friedman, Michelle Collins, Colleen Colbert, Sheila Jardine and David Beisel, Ann Kuehner, Carol and Chuck Mutterperl, Tony and Sally Sapienza, and Joel Weinberger have tolerated unreturned phone calls and/or e-mails, broken engagements, and a general lack of presence. I thank you all for sticking it out with me. I am back.

Finally, this book would not have been possible without the loving nourishment, endless patience, and quirky sense of humor of my family. My delightful new daughter, Mollie, was kind enough to nap consistently for 2 hours each afternoon so Mommy could head for the computer, and she went off to bed at night with little complaint, allowing her mom to get another hour or so of writing in at night. Someday she will know how much that meant. My stepson, Dan, is proud that his stepmom is a writer and was respectful of my writing efforts during his visits. His decency, generosity of spirit, exceptional sense of humor, and kindness to me are continuous sources of joy in my life. My Bosnian stepson, Igor Ibradzic, teased me unmercifully, usually at times when I needed a break, and generally brought quick wit, love, and zaniness to my life during the writing of this book. Finally, the center of my life, my husband Dennis O'Dea, just was there and there and there. He is my love, my partner, my best friend. Thank you, O'Deas.

Joan E. Sarnat

We develop our intellectual interests in the context of relationships, sometimes without being aware of the process. It was not until after I had published my first paper on supervision that I became (consciously) aware that my mother had written a paper on that very topic (R. Sarnat, 1952)! I am grateful to her for stimulating my earliest interest in psychoanalysis, as well as to my father for showing me, by example, the importance of making a contribution to knowledge.

I especially want to express my thanks to my coauthor, Mary Gail, for her initiative in seeking me out as a collaborator. Her unwavering belief that together we had something to say that needed to be said, her facility with and depth of understanding of relational theory, and her willingness to take personal risks by disclosing honestly and fully her own experience of the work inspired and motivated me throughout. Her capacity to pursue our intellectual task while simultaneously becoming a mother amazed and astounded me. Mary Gail, I will be forever grateful for this opportunity to work with you.

Thanks go to Kitty Moore at The Guilford Press, who welcomed and encouraged our project when it was hardly more than a gleam in Mary Gail's and my eyes, and to Jim Nageotte, who took over the project from Kitty. With tact and respect, Jim helped us to hone the book into a more focused and succinct final product, Thanks as well to Jonathan Slavin, Irwin Hirsch, and Sandra Buechler, who all read our first draft and helped us to refine it. And special thanks to Charles Spezzano, who challenged me to make sure that the book set up no "straw men," and to Sue Elkind, who in offering her response to our draft proved once again to be the "quintessential container."

Thanks are also due to the departments of clinical psychology where I learned so much about the process of supervising: The University of Massachusetts, Amherst; Antioch New England Graduate School; and The Wright Institute. I am especially grateful to David Singer, who helped me to begin teaching and writing at Antioch, and whose process-oriented approach to case conference lent support to my own thinking about both case conference and supervision.

My first supervisor at the University of Michigan, Edward Bordin, now deceased, served as a lasting model of the emotional qualities that a supervisor can bring to a beginning psychotherapist, and of the importance of those qualities. Thanks also to my many other supervisors over the years, to the supervisees who have often taught me as much as I have taught them, and to my coparticipants in peer supervision groups, who have explored with me, in a setting of mutual disclosure, the emotional depths that underlie the supervisory process. The colleagues, supervisees, and supervisors who allowed me to use their sometimes quite personal material to bring this book to life all deserve special appreciation.

Thanks also to Jane Burka for joining me in teaching and learning about supervision, and for blazing the trail to The Psychoanalytic Institute of Northern California (PINC). Particular thanks to the vibrant intellectual community at PINC who have exceeded my expectations for a comparative psychoanalytic education. My supervisors, teachers, fellow candidates, and analyst at PINC all played important roles in supporting the development of my thinking about supervision, as well as my confidence in that thinking.

Sincere appreciation to Susan Kolodny for offering me wise counsel, and for setting a fine example of how to write—and take pleasure in writing—a first book. And warmest thanks to Julie Friend, who has been a friend indeed through the stressful stretches of the last several years.

And finally, I want to acknowledge three very important men in my life: my husband, David Hoffman, and my sons, Jascha and Michael. Through the adversities and challenges that beset our family during the past several years, they managed to allow me the space to continue with my work, expressing their pride and interest in what I was accomplishing, while at the same time reminding me that work is only a part of what makes our lives worthwhile.

Contents

THE SUPERVISORY RELATIONSHIP

Introduction

From writing this book, we have come to appreciate the challenging position of supervisees who are the pivotal points in at least two, and usually three, relationships—therapist to a patient, supervisee to a supervisor, and patient to a therapist. We also find ourselves further understanding the possibilities and challenges facing supervisors working within this complex matrix of relationships that are entwined and mutually influential, yet remain distinct from one another. We hope that the reader, too, will gain an enriched appreciation of the complexities of the supervisory relationship.

All psychoanalysts and psychodynamically oriented clinicians, as well as most other mental health practitioners, spend many hours learning the practice of psychotherapy by discussing their clinical work with supervisors. Yet despite the centrality of supervision in the training of psychotherapists and psychoanalysts, there is a relative paucity of literature on the subject. There are, to our knowledge, six comprehensive, originally authored books (Dewald, 1987; Ekstein and Wallerstein, 1972; Fleming and Benedek, 1966; Jacobs, David, and Meyer, 1995; Langs, 1979, 1994) and one edited book (Wallerstein, 1981) on psychodynamic supervision written from traditional ego psychological, or at least decidedly nonrelational perspectives. All are excellent treatments of the supervisory process but they do not fully address the needs of psychodynamically oriented clinicians who subscribe to contemporary relational theories of the structure of mind, health, pathology, and treatment.

Two edited volumes (Caligor, Bromberg, and Meltzer, 1984; Rock, 1997) view supervision as a relationally mediated endeavor, and

1

a third edited volume (Lane, Ed., 1990) in part does so as well. Their contributors generate a variety of perspectives on a number of important supervisory topics such as parallel process, impasses in the supervisory relationship, and the evaluative aspect of supervision. Because they are edited volumes, however, these books do not provide a comprehensive, integrated model of all facets of the supervisory encounter.

These 10 books represent the library known to us of notable books on psychodynamic supervision. When one considers the vast compendium of volumes on topics such as transference and countertransference, treating the borderline patient, disorders of the self, and projective identification, to name a few psychoanalytic topics, one is stunned at the relative neglect of supervision in the psychodynamic literature. In part, this stems from an apparent belief among many clinicians that the ability to supervise is a natural outgrowth of career development, and that it suffices to "do unto others what was done unto oneself" in the course of training. This book, therefore, fills what we view as a significant gap in the literature by providing a unified model of the supervisory relationship built on contemporary relational theoretical paradigms of the mind and of psychoanalytic treatment.

As theories of mind, development, health, pathology, and treatment have changed, especially over the past two decades, models of supervision have not similarly evolved. Theoretical and technical approaches to treatment have moved away from emphasizing drives and drive-related, intrapsychically originating structures of the mind as the seat of an individual's psychological functioning. Today, more and more clinicians see internalized relationships as the key structures of the personality. Interest among many psychodynamic clinicians therefore has shifted from the interpretation of drive-mediated, intrapsychic, usually linguistically encoded material, to elucidation of usually unconscious patterns through which patients continue to enact vital relational configurations originally formed in early relationships and elaborated over the course of development. In treatment, therefore, insight conveyed to the patient by a neutral, relatively nonparticipating, "blank screen" therapist is no longer privileged as the road to cure. The barrier between conscious and unconscious is viewed as dynamic, and insight is understood as the patient's increased ability to formulate experience under auspicious interpersonal conditions. In addition, contemporary relational theory acknowledges dissociation, as well as repression, as an important mechanism organizing psychic material.

In relational approaches to psychoanalysis, it is assumed that therapist and patient enact and gradually make explicit the heretofore implicitly detected internalized relational world of the patient, especially aspects of that world that have been repressed or dissociated. Relationship and experience are privileged as transformational, while cognitive insight, although still a part of treatment, is deemphasized as the sine qua non of growth and change. Greenberg (1996) summarizes this position by saying, "What matters most in treatment is the creation and recreation of a range of experiences, enacted in the new context of the patient–analyst relationship. Putting things into words . . . while important, is secondary to the thing itself, the lived experience" (p. 201).

One would expect that such a radical shift in models of mind and treatment would generate analogous revisions in paradigms of supervision. Surely, a relational paradigm of supervision should have come to stand beside one in which the patient's dynamics and appropriate technique are the primary, and sometimes the only, legitimate topics of discussion between supervisor and supervisee. And, indeed, many writers cited in this book have produced journal articles or book chapters suggesting that the theory and practice of supervision would profit from greater symmetry with contemporary approaches to treatment. This book, however, provides the first descriptively detailed contemporary model of supervision, one that emphasizes that the process of supervision must be in some way analogous to the treatment approach advocated by the supervisor. In other words, the supervisory medium should convey the message the supervisor is trying to teach.

Although we are invested in *our* relational model of psychodynamic supervision, we are aware that there are many ways for supervisor and supervisee to engage successfully in a venture devoted to the supervisee's professional development. One of the tenets of our particular supervisory paradigm, in fact, is that the supervisor and the supervisee uniquely co-construct every supervisory relationship. Therefore, we invite readers to use this book as a point from which to depart and deviate. Our primary goal is to stimulate readers to question consciously their perhaps unconsciously entrenched approach to supervision in order to formulate a working model of supervision consistent with their theory and practice of clinical work.

Throughout this book, we illustrate our theoretical points with detailed supervisory vignettes. Some are taken from our own experiences as supervisors and as supervisees; others have been shared with us by colleagues who permitted us to use their material; still others are composite representations of our work with several supervisees and supervisors. In all cases, identifying data have been altered to disguise patients and colleagues. Except in one case, the vignettes are not verbatim transcripts but, rather, are narratively meaningful condensations of supervisory events and are designed to amplify our theoretical positions with admittedly biased selections of experience. We recognize that they therefore do not always present fully the multiple facets and complexity inherent in most clinical and supervisory situations.

When not describing a specific vignette, we address gender in this book by using male and female pronouns arbitrarily throughout the text. In other words, we speak of "him" about half the time and "her" about half the time when discussing supervisors, supervisees, or patients. We find this less distracting than using "his/her" or "s/he" each time we refer to gender.

Throughout the writing of this book, we have been dedicated to "putting our money where our mouths are" by engaging in a process of mutuality and negotiation, and shared power, authority, and vulnerability. We believe that collaboration of any kind is most effective when the members of the dyad focus on the vicissitudes of their relationship as it develops and changes over time. Therefore, as collaborators on this writing project, we have come to know much about each other—as analysts, thinkers, writers, and people—and have spoken to each other about ourselves and about each other in very meaningful ways.

Relational processes thus molded this book at every stage of its development. As coauthors, we warmly encouraged each other's imaginative output and, at the same time, each risked conveying from time to time disappointment in and disagreement with the other's work. In this way, our professional development has been enhanced profoundly through both the exchange of ideas and the process of mutually stretching our conceptualizations of supervision. As we became immersed in working on the book, we each also reacted transferentially and countertransferentially to the other's real and imagined critiques, and to received and anticipated responses to our work from supervisors, supervisees, and other professional colleagues. Consistent with the spirit of the relational model of supervision proposed here, we engaged with each other in mutual discussion of our fears, hopes, fantasies, and uncertainties about the work we produced. And so we have grown personally as well as professionally through coming to know each other better and the self that the other holds in mind. All in all, we are content that the medium of our coauthorship is consistent with the message delivered in the following chapters.

We developed our interests in relational theory and in supervision in somewhat different ways.

Joan began her training immersed in ego psychology as a doctoral student in Clinical Psychology at the University of Michigan and as a postdoctoral student at the Mount Zion Department of Psychiatry in San Francisco; at the same time that she was involved in running groups in Ann Arbor within a "counterculture" that valued egalitarianism, authenticity, and transparency. This "double life" in the 1970s led her to develop both a respect for and an ongoing critique of ego psychology. When relational thinking began to gain more theoretical prominence in the 1980s, it offered her a way to integrate aspects of those two worlds. Later, her training in a comparative psychoanalytic approach at The Psychoanalytic Institute of Northern California helped to further clarify her views, which continue to be broadly integrative. Joan values the interplay of relationship and understanding in the psychoanalytic process, and seeks to honor both in her writing about supervision.

Mary Gail, on the other hand, completed both her doctoral and postdoctoral training at the Derner Institute for Advanced Psychological Studies at Adelphi University, Garden City, New York, long a bastion of object relational and interpersonal thought and interest in what historically has been termed preoedipal pathology. Thus, Mary Gail's movement toward contemporary relational psychoanalytic approaches was a natural extension of her training. In addition, her work with survivors of psychological trauma, particularly childhood sexual abuse, convinced her that experience—especially the experience of a new relationship with an analyst, with whom both regressive and progressive relational paradigms can be enacted and then made explicit—is the primary mutative factor in treatment. Her collaboration with Jody Messler Davies in writing *Treating the Adult Survivor of Childhood Sexual Abuse* (1994) helped her crystallize her views on a relational approach to psychoanalytic treatment.

Joan's specific interest in supervision arose first from her sense of the inadequacy of some of her prior experiences of being supervised. In particular, she was affected by an extended consultative relationship with a psychoanalyst of worldwide reputation, who wrote with nuance and depth about analysis as an intersubjective process, but who was unable to approach supervision in the same way. When difficulties emerged within both the therapeutic and supervisory relationships, this supervisor was unwilling to address them, and the supervision came to an unhappy and premature end. This experience motivated her to learn more about supervision, especially as she became more involved in supervising.

A second, important context for Joan's work on supervision was her experience a number of years ago supervising five psychology graduate students over the course of a full year, and meeting with them in a weekly case conference as well. Because of the structure for training in this program, one of Joan's supervisees, an advanced graduate student, was also asked to provide an additional hour of supervision each week to the four less advanced students, and then to present her supervisory work to Joan in a weekly consultation hour. The very nature of this educational structure confronted Joan with the different impact that her own and her advanced graduate student's psychologies made in cocreating their unique supervisory relationships with each of the other four supervisees. For Joan, it was sometimes hard to believe that a supervisee and her work could seem so different in the two different supervisory relationships. Joan's first paper on supervision (J. Sarnat, 1992) as well as her continuing interest in conceptualizing supervision from a relational perspective (J. Sarnat, 1997, 1998), stemmed from that fascinating exercise.

Mary Gail's interest in the supervisory relationship, like Joan's, grew out of a disappointing supervision. As an analytic candidate, Mary Gail chose a supervisor noted for his keen appreciation of the transference and countertransference matrices developing in treatment, and for his skill in analyzing the nuances of the therapeutic relationship. In supervision, however, this supervisor took a studiously didactical approach. During the supervisory year, Mary Gail became increasingly frustrated by her supervisor's apparent disinterest in the vicissitudes of his relationship with her. At the end of the year, she talked with him about her reactions to their work together. He responded with openness, integrity, and an interpersonal availability that, in Mary Gail's perspective, had been absent during the supervision. At this point, the supervisor became the supervisor Mary Gail had hoped for in the first place, so much so that they eventually published papers on their unique conceptualizations of their supervisory work (Frawley-O'Dea, 1997a; Hirsch, 1997).

This particular supervisory experience evoked in Mary Gail considerable reflection about the congruence between the supervisory process and the process of analytic treatment being taught. She realized that most supervisors were content-consistent—they taught the supervisee to attend to the data they considered to be important in psychoanalytic treatment. It seemed to her, however, that many, if not most, supervisors were not process-consistent: There seemed to be little analogy between the way in which they conducted analytic treatment and analytic supervision. It was especially surprising to realize that even when supervisors taught supervisees to pay exquisite attention to the nuances of the analytic relationship, they did not engage similarly with the supervisee to address the complexities of the supervisory relationship.

Over the next few years, as Mary Gail became a supervisor herself, she began to develop a theoretical paradigm of supervision (Frawley-O'Dea, 1997a, 1997b, 1997c, 1998) that emphasizes greater symmetry between *what* is taught in supervision and *how* it is taught within the supervisory relationship. Her interest in supervision as a relationally mediated endeavor has grown from there into the current collaboration with Joan.

In order to present a thoroughly delineated contemporary relational conceptualization of supervision, our book covers the following topics.

Chapter 1 offers a historical perspective on psychodynamic supervision. Using Sigmund Freud and Sandor Ferenczi as point and counterpoint "fathers" of classical and relational approaches to psychoanalytic theory and practice, we set in relief convergent and divergent aspects of their respective models and trace their influence on clinical training. We also embed the history of supervision in the wider politics of power characterizing the first one hundred years of psychoanalysis.

In order to locate our relational model of supervision in a broader context, we consider the range of psychoanalytic approaches to supervision in Chapter 2. We also try to help readers position themselves in terms of their current, perhaps not fully articulated, model of supervision. In this chapter, we consider the relationship between the theory of mind and treatment taught by the supervisor, and the paradigm of supervision employed. Finally, we define three distinct models of supervision and three dimensions along which these and all models of supervision can be compared.

Narrowing the context for the model of supervision offered in this book, Chapter 3 begins with a review of contemporary relational psychoanalytic theory. Then, we describe in detail our relational model of supervision, illustrating major theoretical points with extended vignettes. It is in this chapter that we begin to delineate supervision as an endeavor embedded in the dyadic relationships formed by the supervised patient–supervisee and the supervisee–supervisor. Here, we propose a model of supervision in which ever-deepening elaboration of these relationships and their mutual influence is central to the supervisory endeavor.

Concomitant with the development of contemporary relational models of treatment has been a shift in the conceptualization of power and authority in the analytic relationship. Traditional paradigms of psychoanalysis rested on the assumed power of the analyst to interpret the contents of the patient's mind. Similarly, supervisors historically relied on assumed authority to teach trainees the theory and practice of psychoanalysis and psychodynamic psychotherapy. In more contemporary models of the psychoanalytic relationship, power and authority are negotiated and shared to some extent by patient and therapist. While there remain necessary and valuable asymmetries between the members of the analytic dyad, there is greater mutuality and egalitarianism than in previous treatment approaches.

In Chapter 4, we illustrate how our relational model of supervision emphasizes a similar sharing of power and authority while at the same time acknowledging important asymmetries between supervisor and supervisee.

Chapter 5 further presents a relationally mediated view of particular issues of power and authority, including the evaluative component of supervision, the supervisor as representative of the wider professional community, the issue of sexual boundaries within supervision, and the influence of gender on the supervisory process.

Regression, the tendency for someone to revert to more primitive or developmentally earlier modes of thinking, feeling, and relating, is a common component of the therapeutic process. According to traditional paradigms of psychodynamic treatment, only the patient was expected to regress, while the analyst maintained a mature, observational stance. Contemporary psychoanalytic theories emphasize that, often, both patient and analyst have regressive experiences through which much can be learned about both the patient's inner life and the transference and countertransference matrices at play in the treatment dyad. The role of regression in the supervisory process has not been explored extensively because, in general, both supervisor and supervisee have been discouraged from acknowledging and examining regressive experiences emerging in supervision.

In Chapter 6, we extend contemporary clinical perspectives on the value of regressive phenomena to explore their place within the supervisory dyad. These phenomena, when welcomed into the supervisory milieu, frequently provide useful information about both the supervised case and the vicissitudes of the supervisory relationship.

One hotly contested issue in the supervisory literature is the extent to which it is appropriate, or even inevitable, to combine teaching and "treating" within the supervisory encounter. In discussing this book with other professionals over the past few years, it is clear that the teach/treat boundary, as it is termed in the literature, evokes more anxiety in supervisors and supervisees than any other topic related to psychodynamic supervision. It is our position on the teach/treat issue, described and illustrated in Chapter 7, that when the supervisory dyad accepts that transferences and countertransferences—in the supervised treatment and in supervision—are the mutual constructions of the members of each dyad, and that, further, the relational vicissitudes of each dyad are influenced by the other one, it cannot explore these phenomena adequately without addressing the psyches of not only the supervised patient, but also the supervisee and, often, the supervisor as well. Thus, it is impossible to birfurcate completely teaching and "treating" in the supervisory endeavor; rather, supervision becomes itself an analytic process in which these historically defined and demarcated activities inevitably are blurred. The challenge then becomes to delineate a relational model of the teach/treat issue in which "treating" remains indentured to the primary task of facilitating the supervisee's professional learning and development. In this chapter, we describe the general parameters of such a relational approach and then apply the model specifically to supervision with supervisees who are in concurrent treatment, who never have been in treatment, and who have been but are not currently in treatment. Because of the keen interest in this facet of the supervisory relationship, the chapter is particularly replete with illustrations of our model at work in various supervisory dyads.

Another much debated issue in psychodynamic supervision is the extent to which the relational themes of the supervisory dyad legitimately and usefully can be viewed as influenced by parallel process phenomena, defined as the enactment within supervision of key, usually unconscious, aspects of the treatment relationship. In Chapter 8, we present what we think is a unique construction of parallel process. First, we demystify the idea of parallel process by illustrating that it is, in fact, a relational phenomenon that occurs every day in many extratherapeutic relationships. Then, insisting that parallel process is a two-way street through which relational constellations originating in any one dyad may parallel into the other, we delineate several configurations of parallel process.

Supervision is not always a dyadic venture; often, supervision takes place in ongoing supervision groups or in more time-limited case conferences. In Chapter 9, therefore, we develop a contemporary model of case conference. In our approach to individual supervision, the supervisory relationship plays a central role. So too, our model of case conference proposes that group process influences the group's experience of and comments about the presented case, and therefore should be explored within the supervision group. In order to do this successfully, an understanding of groups and psychoanalytic group theory is essential. Here, Bion's ideas about group dynamics are particularly relevant. Much of the relational model of individual supervision presented in earlier chapters applies to our view of case conference, including our perspectives on the value of compatibility between the medium of supervision and the message of the treatment approach advocated by the supervisor, on shared power and authority, on the potential importance of regression within supervision, on the teach/treat issue, and on parallel process.

Unless supervision takes place within the supervisor's private practice, it is sponsored and therefore influenced by an institute, academic department, clinical training program, hospital, or clinic. The relational patterns and power politics at work in the larger organization can either facilitate or impede the safety and freedom of the supervisory dyad. Even when the consultant or supervisor is in private practice, the relational patterns of politics reflected in the wider professional community may well come into play.

In our Conclusion, we examine the potential impact of the organization in which the supervision takes place on the ability of the supervisor and supervisee to work from the relational perspective suggested here. We also discuss the mutual influence of the organization in which supervision takes place and the wider psychoanalytic community.

And so we invite the reader to engage with our approach to supervision, hoping—to paraphrase T. S. Eliot (1942)—that each reader ends her exploration of this book knowing the familiar place of supervision for the first time or in some new way.

CHAPTER 1

Historical Perspectives on Psychoanalytic Supervision

As late-20th-century writers influenced by postmodern philosophical trends, we approach this chapter on the history of supervision by acknowledging its perspectival foundation. This is a constructed historical narrative about the origins and progress of psychoanalytically oriented supervision, intended to orient the reader to major themes about knowledge, power, and authority in the development of psychoanalytic supervision over the past one hundred years. Of necessity, we propose a specific slant on history. The history of psychoanalytic supervision as we understand it and our own model of psychoanalytic supervision exist in dialogue, each informing the other. In turn, our particular rendition of the history of supervision inevitably will influence the reader to engage with the chapters that follow through a particular view of psychoanalytic supervision and its historical, thematic underpinnings.

Psychoanalytic supervision was born and has developed within the larger psychoanalytic culture that, of course, has been embedded in and reflective of wider social–political–cultural trends at work, primarily in Europe and the United States, over the last century. To grasp the historical course of psychoanalytic supervision, particularly regarding the themes of power, knowledge, and authority, we must begin at the beginning, with Freud and his classical psychoanalytic theories.

FREUD AND THE CLASSICAL MODEL
OF PSYCHOANALYTIC THOUGHT

In discussing Freud, we acknowledge that Freud the actual figure has been supplanted over the past century by a variety of metaphorical Freud's, each claimed as progenitor of this or that school of thought. Until quite recently (Aron, 1996; Mitchell, 1988), and with some exceptions (Balint, 1968; Fairbairn, 1944; Sullivan, 1956), most psychoanalytic thinkers were determined to position their theories as having descended directly from what Freud said, what he meant to say, or what he would have said had he lived longer! Still, the most Freudian Freud, one more narrow and less contradictory than the actual, quite complicated and complex man, is represented by contemporary classical psychoanalysis. It is this rendition of Freud and his theories that, over the years, has defined the "Other" among interpersonal, object relational, self psychological, intersubjective, and contemporary relational analysts. It is this metaphorical Freud's canon from which all other schools of psychoanalysis deviate, and in relation to which each school's proponents seek to structure their ideas.

In referring to "classical analysis," we describe some trends in classical theory that, although certainly not characterizing the practice of all analysts who consider themselves "Freudian," generally have been presented as part of the classical theoretical stance (Arlow and Brenner, 1964; Brenner, 1982; Eissler, 1953; Fenichel, 1941; Gray, 1990; Rangell, 1968, 1981) and that substantively differentiate that school of thought from contemporary relational theories.

Classical analysis is defined here as a one-person model of clinical work, with power, knowledge, and authority resting primarily with the analyst. In our understanding of classical theory, it is assumed that a relatively healthier, more fully analyzed, more completely conscious analyst takes on a patient who is a relatively sicker, more conflicted, less conscious individual. Furthermore, it is a given that the analyst has the knowledge and authority to interpret to the patient the contents and mechanisms of his unconscious that become evident to the analyst through the patient's free associations. Verbal interpretation is, in fact, the main currency of this analysis. Transference manifestations are assumed to be intrapsychically motivated and wholly constructed by the patient. The analyst is a neutral recipient of the patient's fantasies and projections. Furthermore, the analyst is considered able to observe competently and translate into conscious awareness for the patient that which has been observed. A patient's doubts about or disagreements with the analyst's offerings most often are viewed as resistance to accepting the knowledge the analyst has to convey.

Some contemporary classical analysts may legitimately object that the classical approach delineated here represents a presentation of "classical" analysis that is outdated and caricatures contemporary thinking and technique. They would argue that it does not, therefore, adequately reflect their own current work with patients or with supervisees (Aron, 1996). Any summary statements about a given clinical approach, of course, portray an archetype devoid of the uniqueness and vitality of any particular analyst at work. We recognize that contemporary classical analysts differ as much from one another as do analysts from any school of thought. Classical theory, however, whether or not followed fully by a given practitioner, has unquestionably influenced psychoanalytic training and supervision in a particular direction and continues to do so to some degree. It is significant to us, for example, that, as recently as the 1990s, one of us (Frawley-O'Dea) was taken to task in her psychoanalytic training program by a senior analyst for allowing a patient to use her first name. Addressing an analyst by anything other than "Doctor" was considered by this analyst to be interpretable resistance under all circumstances. Of course, the way any patient addresses her analyst is significant and can express a multitude of meanings; just as the way in which the analytic dyad arrives at a decision about how each will address the other is significant and can mean many different things. There is much room here for enactment, resistance, counterresistance, transference and countertransference, gender and other politics, and so on. What is striking about this example is the senior analyst's assumption that there is only one acceptable way for every patient to address every therapist, and only one explanation for deviation from that aspect of the frame. The positivist assumptions about knowledge, power, and authority inherent in classical theory can be detected in psychoanalytic supervision as well, as practiced first by Freud and handed down through generations of analysts.

THE FREUDIAN TRADITION
IN PSYCHOANALYTIC SUPERVISION

"Supervision" began informally in 1902, incorporated into Wednesday night meetings at Freud's home. The Wednesday Night Psychological Society consisted of laymen and physicians interested in psychoanalytic theory and practice. Members presented papers on various subjects and sometimes discussed case material. Freud was the unquestioned authority of the group. Max Graf, for instance, states that "the last and the decisive word was always spoken by Freud himself" (in Gay, 1988, p. 174).

Freud insisted on his position of authority about what could be known and accepted within psychoanalysis. Although he welcomed divergence and disagreement, it was only up to a point, and he determined what that point was. Understandably defensive about protecting the fledgling field of psychoanalysis from its many detractors, Freud demanded doctrinal consistency from early "supervisees" and agreement with his particular vision of psychoanalysis, which to him was the only true vision. In a 1913 letter to Ferenczi, for instance, Freud asserts, "We are in possession of the truth; I am as sure of that as I was fifteen years ago" (in Brabant, Falzeder, and Giampieri-Deutsch, 1993, p. 483).

Convinced of the parameters of psychoanalytic "truth," Freud, the first supervisor, initially welcomed and later discarded a number of bright but challenging early analysts who persisted in disagreeing with various notions considered by Freud to constitute psychoanalytic dogma. When Freud ousted these early "supervisees," he did so with a vengeance, as public and private correspondences indicate (in Brabant et al., 1993; in Gay, 1988; in Jones, 1961). Freud once cherished each of these early analysts/"supervisees," including Adler, Jung, Stekel, and Ferenczi, but each invoked his wrath and *ad hominem* denunciation when he seriously deviated from Freud's theories and practices.

We may note that Freud's approach to "supervising" his followers is consistent with the classical psychoanalytic model of treatment as just defined. Here, a senior analyst—Freud—is in possession of knowledge and truth that is to be conveyed downward to the supervisee, who, no matter how bright or creative, is to receive rather than co-construct what becomes known. Viewed in the same way as a patient's resistance, the supervisee's inability or unwillingness to accept the knowledge given by the supervisor is seen as a limitation of the supervisee alone. The supervisor's contribution to any problems in learning, or the possibility of the supervisee adding to knowledge in a significantly divergent way, is not considered. Rather, the supervisor is viewed as a neutral, objective observer of the supervisee and of the case material.

Freud was the first supervisor and thus represents the archetypal supervisor to whom we all maintain a transference of some kind. In his model of supervision, he combined a positivist stance analogous to his model of treatment with a personal insistence on maintaining a position as the ultimate arbiter of truth, knowledge, and power. Although his paradigm of supervision was entrenched by the 1930s and has continued to influence the way in which much psychoanalytic supervision is conducted, another configuration of psychoanalytic treatment and, thus of supervision, was advocated by Sandor Ferenczi early on in the development of psychoanalysis.

A FERENCZIAN MODEL OF PSYCHOANALYTIC SUPERVISION

Sandor Ferenczi of Budapest, at various times, analysand, colleague, cherished friend, and would-be analyst of Freud, like Jung, Adler, and others, was rejected ultimately by Freud. Until his final break with Freud, however, the analytic community held him in high regard for both his theoretical prowess and his clinical acumen. Aron (1996), a modern Ferenczi scholar, asserts, "Ferenczi's contributions to the early history of the psychoanalytic movement were second only to Freud's" (p. 161).

Foremost among Ferenczi's contributions was his focus on the two-person nature of the psychoanalytic relationship. Ferenczi was profoundly aware of the potential impact on the patient of the analyst's conscious and unconscious mind. In 1932, he writes:

> Occasionally one gets the impression that a part of what we call the transference situation is actually not a spontaneous manifestation of feelings in the patient but is created by the analytically produced situation, that is, artificially created by the analytic technique. (in Dupont, 1988, p. 95)

Again that year, Ferenczi writes:

> Subtle, barely discernible differences in the handshake, the absence
> of color and interest in the voice, the quality of our alertness or inertia
> in following and responding to what the patient brings up: all these
> and a hundred other signs allow the patient to guess a great deal about
> our mood and our feelings. (in Dupont, 1988, p. 36)

In these entries from Ferenczi's clinical diary, we see an early
analyst keenly aware of the co-constructed nature of the analytic relational scene. Ferenczi implies the very contemporary idea that the
relational strivings patients bring to treatment interact with the analyst's conscious and unconscious capabilities, affects, fantasies, and
personal relational stance to co-create the resulting transference–
countertransference matrix. Further, Ferenczi expresses concern that
classical analytic technique, in which the analyst remains an absti-
nent, ostensibly blank screen figure, too often recreates an atmosphere of deprivation and hierarchically assumed power that was instrumental in the development of the patient's pathology in the first
place.

Unlike Freud, who felt that analysis was best conducted by an ab-
stinent analyst who refrained from disclosing anything about himself
or his reactions toward a patient, Ferenczi grew to believe that patients
were helped most by an analyst who was willing to engage with them
spontaneously and authentically. Ferenczi privileged as curative the
analytic relationship over interpretation and held deeply that patients
benefited from the analyst's willingness to disclose aspects of his life
and experiences to the patient.

Ferenczi became evermore committed to constructing with the
patient an egalitarian, mutually negotiated relationship in which
power was shared between two participant observers. His profound
commitment to this ideal led him eventually to experiment with two
mutual analyses in which he and each of these patients, R.N. and S.I.,
literally took turns analyzing one another. In retrospect, it is clear that
Ferenczi's mutual analyses of and by R.N. and S.I. pushed the envelope
of mutuality and symmetry too far, in ways that were likely damaging
to patients and analyst alike (Aron, 1996; Balint, 1968; Fortune,
1993). In reaching for the outer edge of mutuality, of distributed power
within the analytic relationship, and of the co-creation of knowledge
and narrative truth, however, Ferenczi bequeathed to us an extreme

counterpoint to the extreme point of the Freudian clinical model, opening the way for succeeding generations of practitioners to delineate and occupy a variety of intermediate positions.

Ferenczi as teacher and supervisor greatly influenced a number of analysts of the subsequent generation, including Alice Balint, Clara Thompson, Therese Benedek, Imre Hermann, and Michael Balint. Michael Balint was Ferenczi's analysand, supervisee, literary executor, and successor, a professional son who felt empowered to carry on, expand, and even critically disagree with his mentor's work, apparently without risking the rejection and devaluation Freud turned toward Ferenczi (in Dupont, 1993).

While we do not have detailed descriptions of Ferenczi's supervision of Michael Balint, we can infer that it had a mutual, nonhierarchical tone, since the latter's subsequent work suggests internalization of Ferenczi's thinking regarding power, authority, and knowledge—or truth—in psychoanalysis. Balint also is sensitive to the potentially constricting influence on the supervisee of the supervisor's abuse of power. Balint (1968) cautions, for instance, that the psychoanalytic candidate is influenced by the personality of the supervisor or training analyst and may consciously or unconsciously accommodate to what is expected rather than finding her own psychoanalytic voice. Balint says that "potentially every child, every patient—or every candidate—can learn any language; which language he actually *will* learn depends on his parents, his therapist—or his training analyst" (1968, p. 93). Here, we see Ferenczi's student, by then a supervisor and training analyst himself, implicitly acknowledging that psychoanalytic supervision is conducted within a relationship to which the supervisor contributes and the course of which she influences. Unlike Freud, however, who felt the supervisor could and should convey *the* truth to the candidate, Balint suggests that there are many strands of psychoanalytic thinking from which a candidate can find and fashion his own theoretical and clinical position:

> All analytical languages must be accepted as peers. . . . Each of them expresses important details of analytic experience, and as long as we cannot translate confidently and reliably the communications expressed in one language into any of the others, we have to tolerate all of them. . . . We have no "primus," only "pares." . . . There are several such analytical languages, each psychoanalytic school having developed its own. (1968, pp. 96–98)

By insisting that each school of psychoanalysis has something valuable to contribute, Balint questions the classical model's assertion that the analyst/supervisor can assume to convey truth and knowledge downward to the supervisee from an authoritarian position. At the same time, Balint appreciates that analytic relationships, clinical or supervisory, do not occur between absolute equals. He recognizes Ferenczi's failure to step into, embrace, and preserve the real and valuable asymmetries inherent in analysis and training. Balint, then, presages a relational model of supervision in which knowledge is imperfectly derived through a mutually negotiated relationship between supervisor and supervisee, in which power, although not equally distributed, is mutually authorized and shared.

SUPERVISION SINCE FREUD AND FERENCZI

Freud and Ferenczi, the two primary voices of early psychoanalysis, provided models of health, pathology, treatment, and thus, supervision that were in many ways located at opposite ends of a continuum regarding power, knowledge, and authority. Over the last one hundred years, as a multiplicity of theoretical schools and training institutes have emerged, models of treatment have adhered more or less to one or the other pole, with great variety and spirited debate, even diatribe, about what constitutes "true" psychoanalysis. Yet until quite recently (Baudry, 1993; Frawley-O'Dea, 1997a, 1997b, 1997c; Harris and Ragen, 1995; Lester and Robertson, 1995; Marshall, 1997; Pegeron, 1996; Rock, 1997; J. Sarnat, 1992; Slavin, 1998; Strean, 1991; Wolkenfeld, 1990), models of supervision have evidenced far less variability than paradigms of treatment and have been closer to the Freudian end of the continuum concerning power and knowledge. In part, this can be attributed to the early ascendancy of a training model designed by Freud's followers from the Berlin Institute. In part, however, the seeming intransigence of a hierarchically constructed supervisory paradigm also reflects the influence of power politics, hearkening back to the beginning of psychoanalysis.

Representing the divergent views of Freud and Ferenczi, their respective followers in the Berlin Institute of Psychoanalysis and the Hungarian School of Psychoanalysis arrived at quite different models of psychoanalytic training. Specifically, the Hungarians felt that the candidate's supervisor, at least his first one, should be his analyst. They reasoned that the candidate's analyst was in the best position to delineate fully and work through with the trainee his countertransference reactions to patients. In turn, they argued that the supervisee would feel safest revealing his work to his own analyst. Clearly, we see here both Ferenczi's concern with enhancing the security of the supervisee and his emphasis on the importance of relational considerations in treatment and, thus, in supervision.

Freud's Berlin Institute, on the other hand, proposed what has come to be known as the tripartite model of psychoanalytic training. Specifically, the Berliners delineated three discrete realms of training: didactic coursework, the candidate's personal analysis, and separate supervision with one or more senior analysts. The Berliners believed that psychoanalytic candidates should be exposed to a variety of viewpoints during their training, a breadth of experience they felt the Hungarian model did not achieve. In addition, as an evaluative component was added to the formal training of analysts, there was concern that the integrity of the analysis would be compromised if analyst and supervisor were the same person. In fact, the Berlin paradigm of training discouraged candidates from attending to the supervisee's countertransference responses. Rather, supervision was to be primarily a didactic exercise, with the candidate's personality and character left exclusively to the purview of the personal analysis (Rock, 1997). Ultimately, the Berlin training paradigm triumphed, and the tripartite training model was institutionalized by the late 1930s.

At the same time that the training of psychoanalytic candidates became more formalized, new theories of psychopathology and treatment, or in Balint's (1968) words, new "psychoanalytic languages," were being formulated in Europe and the United States. As analysts constructed new dialects or spoke with a different accent, often they were subjected to *ad hominem* attacks and labeled as heretics by other analysts who positioned themselves as definers and holders of *the* truth. The infamous Anna Freud–Melanie Klein battles are a case in point.

As the new languages of psychoanalytic theory and treatment themselves coalesced within distinct training institutes, the supervision of candidates became a primary mode of teaching that school's way of speaking psychoanalysis. Often feeling beleaguered by criticism from other psychoanalytic schools of thought, or perhaps unconsciously defensive about their position as "Other," senior analysts used supervision to proselytize and politicize as well as to teach. As early as 1947, Balint (1948) expressed concern that the power politics of psychoanalytic training, begun by Freud, were leading institutes to initiate candidates into sacred dogma rather than encouraging freedom of thought and creative new applications of psychoanalytic ideas. Balint also pointed out that the development of competing psychoanalytic training institutes resulted in an unfortunate emphasis on difference in which programs accused one another of teaching heresy rather than truth.

One result of all this power jockeying has been that, even when a particular institute's theories championed increased mutuality within the analytic relationship, the supervisory relationship often remained frozen in a more hierarchical frame in which power rests almost wholly with the supervisor who conveys knowledge downward to the candidate. As recently as the 1980s, Aron (1996) echoes Balint when he reports that he and fellow postdoctoral analytic candidates at New York University "felt that we were not being encouraged to think for ourselves but, rather, were being asked to choose between party lines" (p. 7) in an institute in which the Freudian track, the Interpersonal/Humanistic track, and a nonaligned Independent track bid to capture the minds and hearts of their trainees. At some other psychoanalytic training institutes, even today, a supervisor must be a graduate of the institute at which she supervises. While this policy offers candidates a deep immersion in the body of theory adhered to by that institute, and while there is significant clinical variability among individual supervisors within any theoretical school, the policy also limits the breadth of theoretical exposure candidates receive and preserves a political hegemony at such institutes, albeit within which other intrafamilial political battles are waged.

The point here is not to criticize this or that psychoanalytic institute. Rather, we want here to set in relief supervision's historical embeddedness in the political power jockeying consciously and unconsciously enacted within every one of the various schools of psychoanalytic thought, each of which often birthed itself by defining its difference from, not its similarity to, some other school of psychoanalytic thought. Consideration of the political and sociocultural aspects of psychoanalytic history thus enriches our understanding of the static nature of supervisory models, even amid the great dynamism and organic evolution of theoretical and treatment models.

CONTEMPORARY TRENDS IN SUPERVISION

Aron (1996) suggests that since the mid-1980s, psychoanalytic thought increasingly has been influenced by postmodern and constructivist philosophical trends, as well as by feminist theorizing, mediated in part by the gender shift within psychoanalysis. Previously a field dominated by male analysts treating mostly female patients, we now operate within a profession in which most practitioners and, certainly most supervisees, are women. In addition to this reconfiguration of the biological gender of psychoanalysis, traditionally rigid constructions of what constitutes male and female have been changing in the direction of flexibility and ambiguity. Aron argues that these contemporary sociocultural emanations profoundly altered the politics of power, knowledge, and authority within psychoanalysis and, in turn, contributed to the development of more relationally mediated theoretical and clinical approaches.

Although these social and political trends, and the concurrent advent of relational theory, in the mid-1980s have begun to thaw traditional notions about the supervisory relationship, the latter often is so embedded in the historical identity and power politics of the institute or organization sponsoring the supervision that change still occurs at a frustratingly slow pace. Slavin (1997) asserts that the shift to a new clinical paradigm "has seemed to affect neither the culture of psychoanalytic training nor the views and practices of candidates about what psychoanalysis is" (p. 813). Writing almost 50 years after Balint (1948), Slavin (1997) sounds much like him when he refers to psychoanalytic training programs of every theoretical school as most similar to the initiation rites of clerical candidates into the dogma of their chosen religion. He argues that a century after its birth, psychoanalysis still is too often taught as truth rather than as possibility.

The similarity of the observations offered by Balint in the 1940s, Aron in the 1980s, and Slavin in the 1990s could engender hopelessness about making substantive changes in psychoanalytically oriented training, including the supervisory relationship. Donnel Stern (1997), however, advises that change often follows a "cultural lag, that gap of months or years that lies between the time a change has begun to occur and the time the culture finds or allows itself the means to represent the change in explicit verbal terms" (p. 55). At this point, the supervisory relationship and the experience of psychoanalytic supervision is just starting to be reconstructed to fit better the changes in psy-choanalytic culture occurring over the past decade. As in models of treatment, paradigms of supervision have been offered (Berman, 1997; Fiscalini, 1997; Fosshage, 1997; Frawley-O'Dea, 1997a, 1997b, 1997c, 1998; Rock, 1997; J. Sarnat, 1992, 1998; Slavin, 1998) that emphasize mutuality, shared and authorized power, and the co-construction of knowledge. It is upon these valuable beginnings, in fact, hearkening back to Ferenczi, that this book builds.

CHAPTER 2

Models of Supervision

Defining and comparing models of supervision can be just as tricky a business as defining and contrasting clinical models (Spezzano, 1998). In both cases, technical overlap between approaches, and variations in technique among practitioners of the same approach, complicate thinking about differences. Despite the complexity inherent in defining supervisory models as distinct entities, generating categories and dimensions, even if they necessarily reify and simplify the infinite variation in individual style, is indeed worthwhile. Creating models that can be compared and contrasted to one another allows us to reflect more systematically on what we do and to locate ourselves within the range of possible models of supervision. In this chapter, we take a look at the full spectrum of models of psychoanalytic supervision.

A TYPOLOGY OF SUPERVISION

In order to facilitate thinking about differences between supervisory approaches, we need to define a set of dimensions along which the various approaches may be readily compared. Any such typology must capture the important dimensions that differentiate supervisory approaches, and its dimensions must be amenable to describing the full range of supervisory styles. Here, we offer a typology consisting of three dimensions, which, although drawing on others (Abrams, 1993; DeBell, 1981; Haber, 1996; Jacobs et al., 1995; Levenson, 1984; Wagner, 1957), offers a breadth and depth that is not characteristic of any of the existing typologies. After defining these dimensions, we apply them to distinguish three distinct models.

25

Dimension 1. The Nature of the Supervisor's Authority in Relationship to the Supervisee

This dimension, which we consider central to describing the supervisory relationship, can be understood as a continuum running between two poles. At one pole, the supervisor views herself primarily as an uninvolved and objective expert who knows what is "true" about the patient's mind and what is "correct" technique. Her authority is based primarily on *knowledge* to be taught. At the other end of the continuum, the supervisor views herself as an involved participant with more expertise, but with no absolute claim to knowing what is "true" about the patient or what is "correct" technique. Her authority is based on a *process* that unfolds within the supervisory relationship. This dimension is not addressed directly in any of the existing typologies of supervision.

Dimension 2. The Supervisor's Focus: The Relevant Data for Supervisory Processing

Many supervisors never stop to consider what they are choosing to focus upon or ignore, or what data they are ruling in or out. Yet these decisions, often made nonreflectively and on the basis of unconscious identification with internalized supervisors, determine what can and cannot transpire in the supervisory situation.

For example, what if the supervisor feels that supervision consists of focusing exclusively on the patient, that is, on his transference and resistance, viewed intrapsychically? If so, the supervisor and supervisee will be limited to discussing the patient's diagnosis, dynamics, and anxieties, and appropriate techniques for treating such a patient. Nothing else will seem possible. The supervisor who assumes that the patient is the primary source of data will also tend to exclude the many occurrences of regressive experience of supervisee and supervisor from the supervisory discourse, and will discuss only the supervisee's secondary process thinking about the patient. By contrast, in other models, the supervisor focuses primarily upon the psychology of the supervisee. In these models, the supervisor considers the supervisee's learning problems and problems about learning, his transferences to supervisor and patient, his anxieties, and the vicissitudes of his self-esteem to be relevant data to be addressed in supervision. Different again are models that focus on the psychologies of all participants in the supervisory situation—that is, the patient, the supervisee, and the supervisor—as legitimate and relevant sources of data. Models that cast this broad net will also consider relevant the organizations and other relational contexts in which these participants are embedded.

It is striking that existing models consistently leave out the supervisory relationship as a possible focus of attention. DeBell (1981), drawing upon Wagner's (1957) earlier work, contrasts supervisory approaches in terms of "whether the focus of the supervisor is predominantly or inflexibly patient-centered, analyst-centered, or process-centered (we hope not supervisor centered)" (p. 41). Here, although "process-centered" is included as a category, focus on the supervisor's own psychology is apparently considered to be self-centered and therefore a negative. Jacobs et al. (1995) also distinguish several different areas of supervisory focus: "patient focus," "interpersonal focus" (e.g., focus on the patient's extratransferential relationships), and therapist–patient "transferential–countertransferential focus." But, again, this typology fails to include a category for focus on the supervisory relationship. Our Dimension 2 very much includes the supervisory relationship, as well as any other relationship that is pertinent to the supervisory and therapeutic dyads, such as the supervisee's relationship with his own therapist, or the relationship of the supervisory dyad to the organization in which it is situated, that may come to be relevant to the supervisory dyad.

Dimension 3. The Supervisor's Primary Mode of Participation

Supervisors view their roles in surprisingly divergent ways. Does the supervisor function primarily as a didactic teacher, an expert on psychodynamics and technique? Or as a Socratic asker of questions or a "Zen master" who refuses to share her own solutions? Is she an interactive and collegial support? Or does she seek to function as a container for supervisee affects and projective identifications? Or as a selfobject? Does she encourage a primarily cognitive or also an experiential engagement in the process of supervision? Is she willing to work with the supervisee's affects, conflicts, and relational themes as these enter into the supervised treatment? How does she understand the teach/treat boundary? And how does the supervisor's chosen mode of participation relate to the clinical theory she is trying to teach the supervisee? This dimension is used to characterize the primary role that the supervisor takes with the supervisee in any or all of these respects. Abrams (1993) and Levenson (1984) each offer a typology that addresses this dimension but, again, leave out the supervisor's function as reflector upon her own participation or as facilitator of the supervisee's similar reflections. We explicitly define this dimension to include all such supervisory participation.

These three dimensions address the most important aspects of the supervisory relationship and can be used to describe a wide range of supervisory models. Although they were intended to stand independently of one another and could theoretically occur in any combination, we have found that most of the supervisory approaches in the psychoanalytic literature can actually be described in terms of three specific clusters of these dimensions. These we consider to be our three primary models of supervision. In addition, the second of these models can be further divided into three submodels, according to the main clinical theory upon which each draws.

Each of these models, of course, represents an "ideal" type, defined for heuristic purposes, and never is used in "pure" form by an actual supervisor in the real world. Although informed by and influenced by her theoretical model, each supervisor of course works in her unique way, adapting to many specifics of the situation, drawing on her unique personality and her knowledge of other theories, and so on. We nonetheless find it useful to differentiate these models as though they were pure entities, because doing so may help supervisors to become more cognizant of how a particular theory of treatment, and therefore supervision, may be influencing their supervisory participation.

THE PRIMARY MODELS OF SUPERVISION

The Patient-Centered (Classical) Model

As we discussed in Chapter 1, the patient-centered model, or classical model, is the model of Freud, and following him, the Berlin Institute. Some supervisors continue to use it today, even though their view of treatment has evolved in a more contemporary direction. Although

MODELS OF PSYCHODYNAMIC SUPERVISION

MODELS	DIMENSIONS				EXAMPLES
	Supervisor's Authority (Chapters 4 & 5)	Supervisor's Focus (Chapters 6 & 8)	Supervisor's Mode of Participation (Chapter 7)		
Patient-Centered (Classical) Model	Supervisor viewed as an uninvolved, objective expert.	The patient's mind and correct technique.	Didactic.		Dewald (1987)
Learning Problem (Ego Psychological)	Supervisor viewed as an uninvolved, objective expert.	The supervisee's resistances or "learning problems" and "problems about learning."	Confrontation, clarification, and interpretation of the supervisee's resistances.		Ekstein and Wallerstein (1972)
Empathic (Self Psychological)	Supervisor viewed as an objective expert, but also as a source of empathic error.	The supervisee's self-states and selfobject needs.	Empathic responsiveness to the supervisee.		Brightman (1984–1985)
Anxiety-Focused (Object Relations)	Supervisor viewed as an objective expert, but also as a receptacle for induced feeling states.	The supervisee's anxieties as evoked by the patient and the therapeutic situation.	Interpretation and holding of the supervisee's anxieties.		Newirth (1990) Jarmon (1990)
Supervisory-Matrix-Centered (Relational) Model	Supervisor viewed as an embedded participant rather than an objective expert.	Relational events, including regressive experiences in the full supervisory matrix.	Participation in and exploration of enactments and relational themes, in addition to other supervisory modes.		Frawley-O'Dea and Sarnat (this volume)

Therapist-Centered Models

this model has already been characterized in the previous chapter, we define it again, in terms of our three dimensions.

In a patient-centered model, *the supervisor's authority* stems from the assumption that she is a relatively uninvolved expert with knowledge of both theory and technique that transcends that of her student. Difficulties that are experienced by the supervisee, or in the supervised treatment, are formulated in terms of the patient's dynamics and the supervisee's technical limitations or countertransference problems. In the case of the latter, the supervisor will likely recommend that the supervisee take the issue to his own treatment. The supervisor is the primary judge of what is "good" theory and technique, and of what is "true" about the patient's mind.

As far as *what the supervisor considers to be relevant data for supervisory processing*, the patient's psychology is primary, and virtually all events transpiring in the treatment will be formulated in those terms. Little attention is paid in this model to the dynamics of the supervisory relationship or to the psychology of the supervisee, both of which are viewed as background only. The goal is for the supervisory relationship to function smoothly, so that it supports the work of understanding and intervening with the patient. When tension develops within the supervisory relationship, the supervisor will attempt to restore the supervisory dyad to conflict-free collaboration as quickly as possible. Processing of conflict within the supervisory relationship is viewed as an inappropriate focus for the supervisor, since it disrupts didactic teaching. The supervisee is expected to maintain as much observing distance from his countertransference reactions to the patient and transference reactions to the supervisor as possible. The supervisor is also assumed to be able to keep her countertransference reactions to the supervisee and to the supervised material from intruding very much on her supervisory participation.

The supervisor's primary mode of participation is didactic, helping the supervisee to understand the patient, and showing him how to respond to the patient's material. Indeed, this model is equivalent to what Abrams (1993) referred to as the "didactic style" of supervision.

Of course, it is not only within the patient-centered model that didactic teaching occurs. In fact, in most approaches, the supervisor functions didactically at least some of the time. Each approach to supervision understands this aspect of the process in its own terms. For example, from a self psychological perspective, a supervisory pair who engage in didactic interaction are making use of an idealizing transference, with the supervisor's expertise idealized in the mind of the supervisee, and with this idealization serving important selfobject functions for the supervisee. From an object relations perspective, such a didactic interaction may be understood as a kind of unself-conscious "playing." From a relational perspective, such interaction could be understood as a time when the needs of the supervisory triad are being addressed through concordant interaction (Greenberg, 1995a), a moment of quiet enactment that may or may not need to be understood as such at a later point.

Strengths of the Patient-Centered Model

This is the model that the classically oriented supervisor is likely to have learned from her own supervisors, and it therefore will come to her quite naturally, and she will feel comfortable and secure in working from it. It is a relatively safe approach for the supervisor, minimizing her anxiety. The rules of technique and the view of the patient's mind are fairly well defined, leading supervisor and supervisee to relax into a sense of relative security that provides refuge from the many anxieties generated by the clinical relationship. This approach therefore works best in the hands of a supervisor who has command of a specific, clearly teachable technique. The supervisee may become quite skilled in working with a supervisor, for example, who teaches the specifics of resistance analysis (Brenner, 1982; Bush, 1995; Gray, 1994). The supervisee learns implicitly from the process of the supervision how to manage a helping relationship with a minimum of visible "intrusion" from the helper's psychology (although, of course, from our perspective, the helper's psychology is always present, whether acknowledged or not). Although parallels thus exist between supervisory and clinical processes, they are not discussed but rather function silently within the supervisory relationship.

This model tends to keep the "temperature" of the supervision low (Jacobs et al., 1995), because the focus of discussion is outside of the room. This can be adaptive at times, especially with an inexperienced supervisee. Lower stress in supervision means less anxiety and more attention for learning. Supervisees who are eager for concrete technical help, and who do not feel safe exposing themselves more personally in a particular training setting, will find this approach a good fit. It will remain viable as long as supervisor and supervisee see eye to eye on the patient and technique, no impasse develops in the supervised treatment, and disruptive affects and enactments do not disturb the supervisory relationship.

Limitations of the Patient-Centered Model

One limitation of this model is its lack of flexibility to adapt to the vicissitudes of human relationships. When the supervised treatment begins to go badly, or the supervisory relationship becomes conflictual, this model does not offer a way of thinking about the problem other than attributing the difficulty to either the patient's psychology or the supervisee's unworkable countertransference. Neither the supervisor's contribution to difficulties nor the supervisee's countertransference issues that might be workable within the supervision are considered. A barriered interaction can ensue at difficult moments, with neither participant really acknowledging his feelings about what is transpiring. The supervisee may retreat into false-self functioning (Eckler-Hart, 1987), keeping his true feelings out of the supervisory situation. The supervisor may do so as well.

Modeling effects do not contribute much to the teaching and learning process, and identification processes are not utilized optimally. Conflictual moments in the supervisory relationship, which could provide an opportunity for the supervisor to demonstrate how difficulties between people can be enacted, reflected upon, and analyzed, are not examined. As a result of this stance, the data available for processing in the supervision are limited.

Supervisors who work from a patient-centered model may also view patient needs as competing with supervisee needs, and feel that consideration of the supervisee's psychology interferes with the supervisor's ethical and moral obligations to the patient. For example, Schecter (1995) recently asserted:

> Ethical considerations require that we assume a patient-centered approach in supervision. . . . When the timing of learning in supervision is patient-centered, a therapist must put aside his or her own fear and anxiety about not knowing, and focus on being helpful to a patient. . . . When a supervisor puts a patient's needs first in supervision, a supervisee learns this central psychoanalytic attitude. This attitude is a professional superego injunction. (p. 167)

Although Schecter's commitment to the patient is laudable, the impact on the supervisee of such an attitude may be stultifying. Like Schecter, Langs (1984) also emphasizes that for the supervisor, the patient's needs for "correct" intervention must take precedence over the supervisee's needs in supervision. Both Schechter and Langs imply that the supervisee's psychology should be kept out of the supervisory conversation, and be taken instead to the supervisee's therapy. But the idea that the supervisee must be "taught" things in supervision that are difficult or impossible for him to accept, without regard to his ability to use the input, because the patient's timing "should" take priority, can be pedagogically problematic. How is the supervisee to learn in an atmosphere that disregards his vulnerability to narcissistic injury, his anxieties, and his timing requirements? How is he to mobilize his own therapy to instantaneously meet his training needs of the moment? In contrast, the supervisor who can hold the subjectivities and needs of the full supervisory triad in mind, rather than privileging only the patient's, will not experience the same sense of competition between them, but will instead consider the tension between them to be just more grist to be processed through the relational mill of the supervision.

The Supervisee-Centered Models

The supervisee-centered models appeared next on the American psychoanalytic scene, starting with Ekstein and Wallerstein's (1972) *The Teaching and Learning of Psychotherapy*, initially published in 1952. In this supervisory approach, for the first time, the psychology of the supervisee becomes as central to supervisory process as the psychology of the patient is to clinical process.

As with the patient-centered model, in all of the supervisee-centered models, *the supervisor's authority* continues to depend to a significant degree upon her being an uninvolved expert. The supervisor's response to difficulties experienced by the supervisee, or within the supervised treatment, depends upon her expert knowledge. The supervisor is viewed as the primary judge of what is "good" theory and technique and of what is "true."

But important contrasts to the patient-centered model emerge along the other two dimensions. As for Dimension 2, *what the supervisor considers to be relevant data for supervisory processing*, in addition to considering the patient's mind, the supervisee's mind is of course a central focus of supervisory attention in each of the supervisee-centered models. As with the patient-centered model, however, little attention is paid to the supervisor's contribution to the process. *The supervisor's primary mode of participation* is no longer that of didactic teacher. Instead, the supervisor works with the supervisee's resistances, anxieties, and selfobject needs in a more direct and analytic way. The supervisor utilizes an experiential approach to the supervisory relationship that is absent from the patient-centered model, engaging the supervisee in a deeper investigation of his experience.

After a latency of 20 years, two other supervisee-centered models followed Ekstein and Wallerstein's model. We will consider each of these three supervisee-centered submodels in turn.

The Supervisee-Centered Learning Problem (Ego Psychological) Model

As ego psychologists, familiar with the value of their clinical model for facilitating therapeutic change, Ekstein and Wallerstein (1972) adapted that model to the supervisory situation, elegantly exploiting the isomorphisms between the two processes. The cornerstone of their approach was the *focus on the concept of resistance, applied to understanding the psychology of the supervisee.* "Resistance" is translated as "learning problems" if it arises in the supervisee's relationship to the patient, and as "problems about learning" if it arises in the supervisee's relationship to the supervisor. Examples of such learning problems and problems about learning include the supervisee who is having trouble presenting material effectively in supervision, or the supervisee who is blocked in empathizing with or understanding something about his patient, or the supervisee who is having difficulty using the information provided by the supervisor to change his mode of intervention with the patient. Here, the supervisor maintains an *authoritative stance*, but *the supervisor's primary mode of participation* shifts from didactic teacher to interpreter of resistance.

Strengths of the Learning Problem Model

Like the other supervisee-centered models, this model addresses two of the major limitations of the patient-centered model: It does not ignore the therapist's psychology, and it allows the supervisor to participate in more than just a didactic way. The supervisor can offer the supervisee on-the-spot help with personality issues that get in his way, rather than relegating those issues to the supervisee's treatment. Like all the supervisee-centered models, this approach is experientially as well as cognitively engaging. The supervisor also offers a valuable model for how the supervisee may work with his patient, exploiting the isomorphisms between the two helping processes by demonstrating how to work with resistances in the supervisory situation. This model is especially appealing for ego psychological supervisors who conceptualize the clinical process in terms of resistance, intrapsychically defined, and who are not interested in considering their own participation in the supervisory process.

Limitations of the Learning Problem Model

As with all supervisee-centered models, this model gives little attention to the supervisor's contributions to the dynamics of the supervisory relationship. This theoretical perspective leads the supervisor to attribute difficulties that arise in treatment to the supervisee's psychology in interaction with that of the patient. Difficulties that arise in supervision are understood primarily in terms of the supervisee's psychology. Because the supervisor is viewed as an objective expert, no other way of conceptualizing tensions is possible. Thus, the supervisee is vulnerable to being made into the container for all of the problems that develop in the supervisory relationship, potentially evoking in him feelings of anxiety, shame, and failure.

Because Ekstein and Wallerstein's (1972) classic book presents extensive vignettes to illustrate their model, it offers the possibility for taking a close-up look at its strengths and limitations. In one vignette, Ekstein and Wallerstein describe the supervisory process that unfolds between Dr. Gabel (supervisor) and Dr. U (supervisee). Dr. U was having significant problems in both the supervisory and the therapeutic relationships, which are summarized by Ekstein and Wallerstein as follows:

> Here is the structure of the problem as they [supervisor and supervisee] came to see it together. In the one situation (doing psychotherapy) Dr. U [the supervisee] was trying to cope with the problem of being too controlling and directive, and of censuring the patient—which the patient perceived as a hostile assault; and in the other situ-

ation (being supervised) Dr. U was trying to cope with the opposite problem of feeling on the receiving end of control, direction, and censure. (pp. 185–186)

Collaboration or "alliance," is highly valued here, as indicated by the explicit emphasis on both parties seeing the problem "the same way." Nonetheless, authority relations are not actually as egalitarian as they might appear. The spotlight rests exclusively upon the supervisee's, Dr. U's, psychology, that is, on his *feeling* of being controlled and censured. What is left out entirely is consideration of the supervisor's, Dr. Gabel's, psychology and how his actual participation with the supervisee may have come into play. Consider another excerpt from this dyad's work, which follows upon Dr. U's observation that he had recently noticed his own reticence to inquire freely into his patient's experience during the therapeutic sessions:

> Dr. Gabel suggested that it might in part reflect a feeling of Dr. U that he had gotten burned too much; often when he did go into a situation with the patient it had come up for critical scrutiny in the supervision as reflecting aggressive and controlling impulses. Maybe Dr. U was just being less spontaneous and more guarded. To this he [Dr. U] assented eagerly . . . he was now so anxious and inhibited about doing things that he had come to regard as bad therapy, and it was getting harder to discuss all this within the supervisory setting. His work was under too much scrutiny. He felt exposed. He was consciously beginning to experience the supervisory sessions only as criticism and censure. And he didn't like that.
>
> Dr. Gabel stated that, perceiving it that way, naturally Dr. U wouldn't like it. And this was the very thing that supervisor and student had been talking about all along, in the same way the patient had so often experienced the therapy—as a hostile assault to be warded off. Dr. U said that there was no analogy in this sense between the two processes. After all, he said, as a beginning therapist, he had made a "contract" to be criticized, so that with him it was amply justified. Dr. Gabel said, "Not really. You made a contract to learn, just as the patient made a contract to be helped, not to be criticized." Dr. U said quietly that he wondered whether he had an inner need always to experience teaching as criticism—and not just here. (p. 185)

Dr. Gabel is sensitive to Dr. U's feelings of being criticized in supervision and concerned about working with those feelings. With Dr.

Gabel's guidance, Dr. U comes to some useful understandings about his unconscious assumptions about the sadomasochistic nature of teaching and learning relationships. This supervisee gains far more understanding of how his own psychology affects his functioning as a therapist and as a supervisee than if his supervisor had remained in a purely didactic mode, limiting the supervisory discussion to the patient's psychology and ways of intervening with the patient. Dr. U is also helped by his supervisor to see the parallels between his own conflict and that of his patient.

However, in our view, the usefulness of this approach is limited by Dr. Gabel's apparent assumption that Dr. U's experience of Dr. Gabel has nothing to do with Dr. Gabel's participation, and is exclusively a product of Dr. U's own mind, in this case, his sadomasochistic trends. What is not considered, because of the era in which this supervision took place, and because the theory of supervision guiding this work does not point in this direction, is the possibility that Dr. U's experience of his supervisor may include elements of accurate perception and actually be an intersubjective product. That is, it is possible that Dr. Gabel may *also* have an approach toward teaching that contributed to Dr. U's experience of him and to his difficulties in the supervisory relationship. Thus, even while the *content* of Dr. Gabel's interventions question his supervisee's masochistic submission to his supervisor ("You made a contract to learn . . . not to be criticized"), the *process* ("Let's both focus exclusively on your psychology rather than on our mutual interaction") could perpetuate that submission.

Dr. Gabel's approach, based on a model that focuses exclusively on Dr. U's mind, also neglects to consider how the supervisory and clinical dyads may reciprocally influence one another, with tensions in the clinical dyad flowing up to the supervisory dyad, and vice versa. The learning problem-centered model does not invite reflection upon the complex interrelations of the full supervisory matrix.

The Supervisee-Centered Empathic (Self Psychological) Model

A second variant of the supervisee-centered model may be called the empathic model. In the 1970s, American self psychologists, following Kohut (1971, 1977), developed this supervisory model from their clinical approach. *The nature of the supervisor's authority* is softened a bit here in comparison to the learning problem-centered model, in that the supervisor is viewed as less of an objective expert. She is understood to make errors in empathic responsiveness, and the supervisee's point of view on his supervisor's empathic errors is explored rather than viewed as resistance. At such moments, the supervisor scrutinizes her own participation from her supervisee's point of view to understand the nature of her failure to empathize with the supervisee. The *primary focus* is on the supervisee's self-states, including challenges to grandiosity that inevitably occur as one begins to treat patients, and depressive reactions to such challenges, and the supervisee's need for the supervisor's empathic responsiveness to cope with such reactions. The supervisor works to understand the supervisee's selfobject and developmental needs, and tries to address them, and works to help the supervisee to understand these needs in his patient. *The supervisor's primary modes of participation* are empathic responsiveness, availability for idealization and mirroring, and the working through of empathic failures in the supervisory relationship.

Examples of this model in the literature are provided by Brightman (1984–1985), and Mordecai (1991). Brightman, for instance, describes a beginning trainee's sense of dejection at not being able to fulfill his self-expectation of fully formulating a patient's difficulties after the first interview. The supervisor responds empathically and also makes himself available for idealization, thus helping to relieve some of the trainee's sense of failure and narcissistic injury. Over time, the supervisor helps the supervisee to work through and relinquish his idealization of his supervisor in a gradual and nontraumatizing way.

Strengths of the Empathic Model

Just as self psychological clinical theory represents an important step forward, from a more exclusively confrontational stance toward the patient via focus on her resistance to a stance that can include more attunement to the patient via a focus on her selfobject needs, so too does the empathic model of supervision represent an important shift in the supervisor's attitude toward the supervisee. This model is particularly helpful with supervisees who struggle with high levels of shame, feelings of failure, or despair about their ability to do the work. In response to their supervisors' empathic responsiveness, their anxiety decreases, and they develop confidence in themselves. They also find themselves able to identify with their supervisor's empathic stance when they are functioning as therapists. Indeed, it might well be argued that all supervisees could benefit from substantial doses of empathic responsiveness and opportunities to idealize their supervisors during the arduous process of becoming a psychoanalytic therapist, and that it is useful for all supervisors to become attuned to the universality of supervisee narcissistic vulnerability.

Limitations of the Empathic Model

Since the supervisor's self-reflective efforts are focused upon the causes of empathic failure from the point of view of the supervisee, the supervisor's separate subjectivity is not considered as such.* Because the supervisor working from this theoretical perspective is committed to participating as a selfobject for the supervisee, understanding of relations between separate objects, including aggressive and erotic transference–countertransference constellations and their accompanying anxieties, may tend to be neglected (Mitchell and Black, 1995). She may also fail to pick up on the complex enactments that can link the supervisory and therapeutic dyads.

The Supervisee-Centered Anxiety-Focused (Object Relations) Model

This third variant of the supervisee-centered model did not appear in the United States until the 1990s, although various object relations theories had already been recognized by American psychoanalysis for more than a decade. In the anxiety-focused model, *the supervisor's authority* depends on her role as expert in helping the supervisee to become aware of and to work with primitive anxieties evoked by the patient and the clinical situation. *The relevant data for supervisory processing* include two specific aspects of the supervisee's psychology. The supervisor pays close attention to the supervisee's unconscious anxieties as they arise in the relationship with the patient and manifest themselves in the relationship with the supervisor, and she attends equally to the enactments that the supervisee brings into the supervision as a result of identification with the patient's internal object world. *The supervisor's primary modes of*

---

*Sloane (1986) and Reams (1994) offer specifically intersubjective versions of this model to which this limitation does not apply.

participation are containment and interpretation of the supervisee's anxiety and enactments. The supervisor helps the supervisee to help the patient by providing a space in which the supervisee can be confronted with and helped to bear the anxieties and unsymbolized experiences evoked in the therapeutic relationship.

Newirth (1990), working from a Kleinian clinical model, classifies the therapist's typical anxieties in Kleinian (Klein, 1946) terms: schizoid anxiety, or fear of being abandoned in the analytic situation; paranoid anxiety, or the loss of boundaries in relationship to the patient (projective identification and de-differentiation of the transference and countertransference); depressive anxiety, or tolerating hatred toward the patient and resulting feelings of guilt. His approach is to clarify and confront these supervisee anxieties as they become evident within the supervision hour.

Jarmon (1990), making use of a more Winnicottian object relations approach, emphasizes "holding" as an important function of the supervisor. He describes the supervisory process as one that involves supervisees' enactments of internalized relationships with their patients. The supervisor's task is to create an environment in which the supervisee feels safe to describe the details of his countertransference experience. Internalized relationships and anxieties thus can be consciously and unconsciously communicated to the supervisor, who holds the supervisee emotionally as these disturbing experiences enter the supervisory dialogue, and then helps the supervisee to symbolize the experiences and to process them.

Strengths of the Anxiety-Focused Model

This model provides real help with, as well as ways of making sense of, emotions that may otherwise feel frightening and confusing to the supervisee, and shows him by example how the process of emotional holding works. Thus, an affectively vital supervisory relationship can develop. Supervisees appreciate their supervisors' sensitivity to and willingness to share the anxieties that are inevitably generated in the therapeutic relationship.

Limitations of the Anxiety-Focused Model

This approach may cause the supervisee to feel unbearably exposed if his anxieties are invited into the supervisory relationship, and then are actively interpreted, rather than merely held by the supervisor. This is of course more likely to happen if the supervisor is focusing on the supervisee's anxieties, to the exclusion of her own, and if the supervisor does not appreciate how she herself may be a source of considerable anxiety for her supervisee.

The Supervisory-Matrix-Centered (Relational) Model

Because we devote the remainder of this book to elaborating this model in detail, we only describe it schematically here, in terms of our three dimensions. In a relational model, *the supervisor's authority* derives from her capacity to participate in, reflect upon, and process enactments, and to interpret relational themes that arise within either the therapeutic or supervisory dyads. She derives less authority from her role as expert on psychoanalytic theory and technique, viewed as objective truth, and more from her ability to process the experience that unfolds between herself and her supervisee. She sees herself as an embedded participant in a mutually influencing supervisory process. *The data that are relevant for supervisory processing* are more inclusive than in the other models. Relational themes are assumed to reverberate between the supervisory and therapeutic dyads, and themes are also expected to enter the supervisory and therapeutic relationships from the organizations in which each is embedded, as well as from the therapist's own treatment. All of this is considered grist for the supervisory mill. In addition, all aspects of the participants' experience, including regressive experience—affects, dreams, somatic experiences—are considered relevant data. *The mode of participation of the supervisor* may include exploration of the many aspects of unconscious engagement of the various participants and the inevitable enactments that permeate the supervisory and therapeutic relationships. The supervisor may participate in a range of ways—imparting information, serving containing or selfobject functions—but always with a relational consciousness and readiness to acknowledge the mutuality of the supervisory interaction. This is a highly experiential approach to teaching and learning.

Since the rest of this volume elaborates what we view as the strengths of a relational model for those supervisors who teach a contemporary approach to psychoanalytic treatment, we do not go into them here. But it may be of use to mention one very real limitation of this approach. The supervisor utilizing this model, aware of the many relational complexities of the supervisory process and the difficulty in defining "effective" technique at any particular moment in a particular therapeutic dyad, may at times find herself nostalgic for the "good old days," when "correct" technique seemed easier to define and therefore to teach. Who *would not* miss the sense of calm conviction that comes from offering what are felt to be clear technical prescriptions? The supervisor working from a relational model may at times offer specific technical guidance to the anxious beginning psychotherapist who longs for concrete help (Josephs, 1990), but she cannot do so without also internally confronting how very much more complicated and uncertain the technical situation really is.

A RELATIONAL MODEL VERSUS ENLIGHTENED ECLECTICISM

As we have pointed out, each of the different supervisory models, including the relational model, has important insights to contribute. Creative supervisors therefore reach beyond their own clinical model at moments to take advantage of insights into the supervisory process that are drawn from other clinical models, if they find them compatible with their own approach. For example, psychoanalytic supervisors of a variety of orientations can benefit from Ekstein and Wallerstein's ideas about working with the defenses and resistances of supervisees, Brightman's understanding of the selfobject needs and vulnerabilities of the supervisee, Newirth's understanding of how to work with deep anxieties in the supervisee, and Jarmon's appreciation of the value of psychological holding of the supervisee, without necessarily considering themselves teachers of ego psychological, self psychological, Kleinian, or Winnicottian theory and technique. Similarly, the insights gleaned from a relational clinical model may be of use to many supervisors who do not exclusively identify with the relational school of psychoanalysis.

   So why not adopt a position of enlightened eclecticism as the ideal approach to supervising and leave it at that? Why advocate for a supervisory-matrix-centered (relational) model in particular? Some supervisors, themselves trained traditionally but influenced by postmodern currents in our field, are already rethinking some of the limiting assumptions of more traditional supervisory approaches and integrating postmodern assumptions into their supervisory work in an informal way (Doehrman, 1976; Pegeron, 1996; Sloane, 1986). In particular, the stance of the supervisor as authoritative expert and the exclusion of the psychology of the supervisor from supervisory attention at moments of conflict and tension have begun to be reconsidered. The resulting hybrid supervisory approaches are, in those specific regards, "relational," or "intersubjective," or "contemporary" and far more effective than more traditional approaches. Yet they may still fall short of offering some of the advantages of a frankly relational model. For us, full understanding of this model can provide a perspective on supervisory process that eclecticism, however contemporary and enlightened, cannot.

For example, without a full understanding of a relational model, few supervisors will appreciate the importance of actively *inviting* supervisees to articulate their experience of the supervisory relationship rather than merely responding when supervisees initiate such discussions. They may not see the reasons for putting so much weight on the supervisor's creation of an environment in which a supervisee will feel able to introduce the issues that are his greatest source of anxiety, that is, issues that involve difficult feelings toward the supervisor. The following illustration shows how this can make a great deal of difference in the way the supervision goes.

Jay, an experienced clinician, was supervised by a contemporary object relations analyst, Lawrence, who did not identify with an explicitly relational approach to supervision. Lawrence focused his comments primarily on the patient and never actively encouraged Jay to talk about his experiences in supervision, although he was clearly an open and nondefensive person, dedicated to developing analytic understanding, in a contemporary sense, and well able to consider his own involvement in processes that unfolded in the supervised treatment and the supervisory relationship.

Jay began to present Tess, a woman in her 30s, whom he had been seeing for several months. Tess was a compulsive woman who suffered from depression and a sense that her relationships lacked depth and intimacy. Lawrence suggested that her inner world was dominated by a struggle between an actively coping but controlling and omnipotent "fix-it self," and a vulnerable "dependent self." Tess frequently invited Jay to join in with her self-improvement schemes, which Lawrence saw as being initiated by her "fix-it self." Lawrence worked hard to help Jay understand the defensive function of those schemes and tried to keep him from colluding with them.

Jay was wary of Lawrence's adversarial attitude toward Tess's "fix-it self," feeling that the "fix-it" part of Tess was a source of needed strength for her, an identification with her "can-do," if compulsive, father that she desperately needed in order to counteract her identification with her depressed and passive mother. In this way, Jay disagreed with his supervisor.

After several months of supervision Jay found Lawrence's view of Tess's "fix-it" self unexpectedly intruding into his work with Tess. He said to her, out of context, "I wonder if you might be concerned that I will want to take away your 'fix-it' self?" As soon as Jay heard himself say this, he recognized that his interpretation was actually not attuned to Tess's anxieties at that moment, but rather expressed his own concern.

Tess immediately and anxiously picked up on the comment. Did Jay bring it up because he *wanted* to take it away from her? Did he think this part of her was bad? Because if he did, they had a problem. She liked that part of herself and needed it, and just wanted Jay's help in taming it a bit—"fixing it" in fact. Having realized his own anxiety, Jay limited himself in that session to exploring with Tess what it would have meant to her if he had indeed intended to take that part of her away.

In the following session, which took place before the next supervisory meeting, Tess provided Jay with an opportunity to work further with the anxiety that he had introduced into their relationship. He was able make contact with Tess's dependent self when she, uncharacteristically, allowed it to surface in that session. When she then asked him again why he had said what he had in the previous session, he acknowledged that a part of him did indeed want to confront her "fix-it self," but contextualized his desire to confront that part of her as part of his wish to stand up for this weaker dependent self that had just emerged. Tess was moved by his explanation, which was certainly a true if not complete one. Jay in turn felt relieved that he had been able to repair the rupture with his patient and to re-create the sense of the two of them as a mutually regulating dyad.

But for Jay, repairing his relationship with Tess was only half the job. After that session, he realized that his comment had been triggered by an unprocessed aspect of his relationship with his supervisor. He understood that, on some level, he felt that to please his supervisor, he *had* to confront Tess's "fix-it" self, and that this sense of pressure had thrown him off balance in his relationship with Tess. It is important to note that Jay's insight into his feelings toward Lawrence emerged *after* he had himself repaired the rupture with Tess and his confidence in his ability to work with her had been restored. Jay, who was an experienced and relatively confident clinician, could not even *think* about the issue, much less bring it up with Lawrence, until he had himself righted things with Tess and thus felt less vulnerable to feelings of shame and humiliation.

Jay did then bring the issue up with Lawrence, although it was frightening for him to do so. Happily for Jay, Lawrence was non-defensive, noncritical, and interested. Jay felt able to spell out his feelings about his supervisor's attitude toward Tess's "fix-it" side, and how he felt those feelings had intruded into his work with her. Lawrence commented that Jay had intuitively picked up on the fact that Lawrence had "some quite aggressive internal objects," and that he realized that he at times might therefore come across as harsher than he intended. But Lawrence also thought that Jay had misunderstood what he actually felt Jay should be *doing* with Tess. They then had a useful discussion about Lawrence's own approach to technique, which, in this case, was to try to connect to the dependent self rather than to try to confront the "fix-it" self. This was, of course, the tack that Jay himself had taken with Tess in the follow-up session, when he had repaired the rupture with her. Jay realized that despite the psychic reality of his feelings of anxiety and difference with his supervisor, in actuality, he and his supervisor saw the technical issue itself quite similarly!

Jay wondered why he had misunderstood Lawrence as he had, and reflected that he, too, had aggressive inner objects that were more than ready to take his supervisor's words and make them into a harsh directive that must be followed precisely in order for Jay to warrant his supervisor's esteem. Lawrence observed that Jay's harshness also represented an identification with Tess's inner world—that *she* felt those kind of pressures to "follow orders" and "take harsh action" or risk the disapproval of her own internal "committee" all the time. When Lawrence made this link, it helped Jay to understand more about Tess's experience. And Lawrence's accepting response helped Jay to create a space within himself for living with and becoming analytically interested in "committee"-like internal objects—his own, his patient's, and his supervisor's.

This supervisor's way of working defies simple classification. Teaching an object relations model of treatment, he was primarily focused on the patient but was also willing to consider the supervisee's psychology and his own when asked to do so by his supervisee. Importantly, his stance toward his own authority was in keeping with a relational model: He was open to hearing and honoring his supervisee's experience of him rather than assuming that his own perspective was the only "correct" one. He thus contributed to the creation of a powerful experience in supervision that modeled the kind of work he was trying to teach his supervisee to do. In all of these ways, he was a flexible and available supervisor who offered many of the qualities of a relational model supervisor. However, in one important way, he did not do so.

Lawrence did not make studying the full relational matrix a priority. He did not invite Jay to discuss his reactions to the supervision, either with a general invitation at the start of the relationship or later, when he sensed subtle tensions developing. Instead, it was left to Jay to initiate the conversation. This Jay could not do until he had independently worked through his difficulty and felt some renewed confidence in himself. A less experienced and self-confident supervisee would probably not have felt free to bring the issue up at all without an explicit invitation from his supervisor. The whole experience would likely have gone unexplored and, as a result, a subtle distance would have developed within this supervisory dyad. The patient might have suffered as well, as her therapist's disruptive identification with a (fantasied) aspect of the supervisor continued to intrude upon the therapeutic relationship. And the supervisee's deeper appreciation of persecutory inner objects would never have developed.

Lawrence did not himself invite the necessary conversation because, despite his openness to Jay's perspective, he did not subscribe to a theory of supervision that sensitized him to the importance of doing so or allowed him to view such conversations as central to the teaching and learning process. Lawrence's theory of supervision, to the extent that he had articulated one for himself—and, in our experience, many supervisors have not yet articulated for themselves a theory of supervision—viewed such conversations as peripheral to the primary task.

By way of contrast, we offer an example of a supervisor who aimed to teach some of the same contemporary object relations understandings of treatment and approached treatment from a comparative psychoanalytic perspective but worked from a more fully relational model of supervision. Consider the subtle but important ways that this supervisor's stance differs from that of the previous supervisor as she takes an active role in inviting discussion of the supervisee's distress.

After several months of work with Esther, a psychology graduate student, her supervisor, Denise, began to sense some tension developing in their relationship. Although on the surface Esther continued to act as if all were well, Denise was not convinced. At the start of supervision, Denise had told Esther that she felt it was very important that they communicate openly and frequently about how Esther was experiencing their work together. In response to her sense of subtle tension, Denise now explicitly asked Esther how things were going for her in their supervision.

Esther responded by tentatively expressing concern about her work with her patient, Caroline, whom she had been seeing weekly for several months. Esther had persisted for the last several weeks in trying to analyze Caroline's request for a referral for antidepressants, rather than just agreeing to provide the referral. Caroline was reacting with intense upset and anger, and putting a great deal of pressure on Esther. Esther had begun to worry that she was hurting Caroline by withholding the requested referral.

At first, Denise had trouble grasping why this issue should be creating tension in their supervisory relationship. Denise recalled that Esther had earlier expressed her preference to analyze Caroline's request, rather than just going along with it, as was common in this brief treatment setting. Esther had felt that to do so would be a repetition of Caroline's father's hurtful ways of treating her—"handing her off to the doctor"—and Denise was impressed with Esther's formulation and supported her decision to stick with it. On the other hand, Denise had no sense that it would be "wrong" for Esther to rethink her position if it did not feel therapeutically useful at present.

Esther, however, acted as if changing her own position would put her in conflict with her supervisor, as if Denise were committed to this unhelpful therapeutic stance. Denise responded by making the supervisory relationship issue explicit, as Esther seemed to experience it: "You must be feeling some doubt about the position I took on this matter with you." She thus accepted Esther's current perception that it was Denise, not she, who was the obstacle to rethinking this particular technical position. Esther then expressed her doubts about her supervisor's counsel with considerable emotion. For Esther, her disagreement with "Denise's position" apparently felt like a frightening challenge to Denise, and an attack on Denise's expertise. She seemed to anticipate that Denise would become defensive and blame her for the difficulties she was having with Caroline. Instead, Denise heard Esther out, and then told her that she was open to discussing the question again. Perhaps there was more that they needed to understand about this difficult therapeutic situation in which Esther found herself.

Esther expressed great relief, saying that she now realized that until this discussion, she had been feeling that she was alone in worrying about what to do with Caroline. Denise's response had made her feel that she could depend on her supervisor to share responsibility for Caroline's distress—that her supervisor would not leave her alone in her anxiety or feelings of failure, or need her to take all of the blame.

After this supervisory hour, Esther was able to go back to Caroline, to hear her out more comfortably, and to consider freshly Caroline's request. In response, Caroline relaxed and acknowledged that she found it useful to talk her feelings through! Caroline did not raise the issue of referral for medication again.

How are we to understand this sequence? Esther was anxious and reluctant to bring up her anger and critical feelings toward her supervisor, whom she viewed at that moment as rigid, misguided, and defensive, and would not have done so without her supervisor's active support. Esther's conflict about expressing disagreement with her supervisor could be viewed as a reaction to her patient's attack on her, as well as a possible expression of Esther's own need to experience an authority as strict and withholding of support. When Esther risked expressing this (fantasied) disagreement, it became possible for Denise to provide her with a model for responding to the expression of distress and anger in a helping relationship. In typical parallel process fashion, Esther succeeded in evoking in Denise the same anxieties that Caroline had evoked in her, anxieties about causing distress to both Esther and Caroline. Esther then could watch Denise grapple with those anxieties. When Denise managed them in a calm and nonretaliatory way, Esther seemed to identify with Denise's ability to bear those anxieties, and brought this enhanced capacity back into her work with her patient.

Just as in the previous vignette with Jay and Lawrence, Esther felt that her supervisor was a source of disruptive technical advice, although in both examples, the supervisors actually felt differently than the supervisees assumed. Both supervisors were accepting, nonde-fensive, and well able to contain the affects introduced by their supervisees. Working from a relational model, however, Denise appre-ciated the importance of actively inviting into the supervisory rela-tionship an undercurrent of tension that could well have been ig-nored, coming as it was from an anxious and eager-to-please beginning supervisee. If Denise had not done so, Esther would most likely have continued to hide her distress, and the stalemate with the patient, ad-dressed merely at a technical level, would likely have persisted. In-stead, Esther was able to get her supervisor's help in processing the re-lational theme that was currently most conflictual in the transference–countertransference in her case.

We have considered the spectrum of psychoanalytic supervisory models in terms of our own typology and have discussed the contribu-tions and limitations of each. We now proceed with a full elaboration of our supervisory-matrix-centered (relational) model of supervision. In doing so, we hope that even clinicians who do not explicitly iden-tify themselves as "relational," but who think about psychoanalytic theory from a broadly postmodern perspective—clinicians like Denise in the previous vignette—will find that this model has something of value to offer them.

CHAPTER 3

A Relational Model of Supervision

Models of supervision developed more or less in tandem with shifts in schools of psychoanalytic theory. For example, supervisors could not delineate a "supervisee-centered empathic model of supervision" without the clinical theories of self psychology serving as a foundation. It was the development of self psychological concepts, such as the individual's need for selfobjects, the self-preserving fantasies leading to idealizing transferences, the importance of empathy in preventing fragmentation of the self, and so forth, that both permitted and directed supervisors to focus on the vicissitudes of their supervisees' self-esteem and the threats to self-coherence potentiated by the supervisory process.

So, too, a relational model of supervision could not be conceived and elaborated until the relational school of psychoanalytic theory was born and attained some measure of maturity. To contextualize our contemporary model of supervision, it is helpful to introduce it with reference to key concepts of relational theory. This treatment of relational psychoanalysis is necessarily schematic. We do not pretend to explicate fully the variations of relational theory, nor do we define areas of disagreement among relational thinkers.* Our discussion of rela-

---

*For more thorough discussions of relational theory, including the ways in which relational thinkers diverge from one another, the reader is referred to Aron (1996); Bromberg (1998); Davies and Frawley (1994); Hoffman (1998); Mitchell (1988); Mitchell and Aron (1999); Pizer (1998); Skolnick and Warshaw (1992); Slochower (1996); Spezzano (1993); and Stern (1997); as well as the library of issues of *Psychoanalytic Dialogues*, the flagship journal of the relational school of psychoanalysis; *Contemporary Psychoanalysis*, the primary journal of interpersonal theory; and *Psychoanalytic Quarterly*—each of which has published many relationally oriented articles.

tional theory may at times appear simplified and idealized, and may portray a unity of thought that cannot, of course, characterize the full range of practitioners in the field. Rather, we are presenting a theoretical archetype, much as we earlier offered an archetype of classical theory, as a basis for building our theory of supervision.

Relational theory assumes that individuals from birth on develop in the context of the relationships that they struggle to engage in and maintain, and from which they attempt to extricate themselves. Like Fairbairn (1943) before them, relational theorists, supported by the infant and toddler research of the past 30 years, see the human organism as object seeking from birth; thus the drive to attach and to relate is the primary drive. Mitchell (1988) puts it well: "The evidence seems overwhelming that the human infant does not become social through learning or conditioning, or through an adaptation to reality, but that the infant is programmed to be social. . . . The very nature of the infant draws him into relationship" (p. 24). In relational thinking, intrapsychic and interpersonal development and realms of psychological functioning emerge and continue to be structured in dialectical tension over the life span. Mitchell again poetically elaborates the interrelationship of the intrapsychic and the interpersonal, saying, "Like Escher's *Drawing Hands*, the interpersonal and the intrapsychic realms create, interpenetrate, and transform each other in subtle and complex manner" (p. 9).

With the privileging of relationship and the emphasis on the inextricable, mutual embeddedness of the interpersonal and the intrapsychic elements inherent in relational theory, relationships become the primary constituents of psychic structure. Mind becomes organized by units of internalized relationships.

Recently, the relationally mediated structuralization of mind delineated by relational theory has been applied by some thinkers (Bromberg, 1996; Davies, 1996; Harris, 1996; Mitchell, 1993; Pizer, 1998) to redefine the entire notion of self. Throughout most of the history of psychoanalysis, developmental and clinical emphases have been on the adaptive nature of a unitary self. Health implied a single self and, therefore, discontinuities of self and, certainly, paradoxically organized self-states functioning in opposition to one another were by definition pathological. As contemporary analysts have been drawn to postmodern philosophical trends, however, the whole concept of a privileged, unitary self has been refuted by some and replaced by a

model of a normative, multiple self-system organized more by dissociative mechanisms than by repressive processes.

Within this contemporary model of self, actually presaged by
Janet (1889), the early Freud (1893), Ferenczi (1932), and Fairbairn
(1944), the individual is seen as constituted by a multiplicity of self-
states. Each self-state represents the experiential precipitate of internalized relationships and includes, according to Davies (1996), a "self-
representation, an object representation, a predominant affective
tone, an experience of somatic body-state, and a level of cognitive organization" (p. 562). Some constellations of self are so fundamentally
reinforced and elaborated during development that they come to reflect for the individual the most familiar experiences of "me." Others,
encapsulating less usual or more disturbing selfobject internalizations
and self-systems, are experienced as alien, confusing, not quite accessible, intrusive, or even hateful and hated states of self.

In health, when the person's developmental experiences have
been, for the most part, good enough, the mind can maintain a dialectic encompassing what Pizer (1996) describes as the paradox between
"mutually exclusive elements which must continue to coexist, even
while negating each other's existence" (p. 502). We like Pizer's deno-
tation of this multiplicity of selves in health as a "distributed self; that
is, a self distributively structured among multiple memorial islands of
relational experience but held integrally by the mind's capacity to
bridge paradox" (p. 503). Here, we have a normative multiple self,
structured through a lifetime of sometimes contradictory relational experiences, psychically constituted through dissociative processes, and
marked often enough by paradox. Furthermore, this self is primarily
motivated to express its variety of self-experiences through relationships with others.

That is health. Not surprisingly, relational theory's understanding of psychopathology derives from the impact and internalization
of relational disappointments or trauma on the developing and mature psyche, and on the individual's intrapsychic attempts to cope
with these phenomena. As health is constituted by the interpenetration of the intrapsychic and the interpersonal, so too is psychopathology. Mitchell (1988) says, "Psychopathology, throughout its
entire spectrum, may be defined in its broadest terms as the tendency of people to do the same painful things, feel the same unpleasant feelings, establish the same self-destructive relationships, over

and over and over" (p. 26). The primary aim of the repetition compulsion, as defined here, is to preserve the individual's attachment bonds to significant figures in her life, as well as to master conflict and to ward off unacceptable self- and other representations. It is both the drearily familiar unpleasant outcomes of repeated pathological relational strivings *and* the inflexibility of the patient's relational repertoire that constitutes psychopathology.

Relational theory emphasizes the active, albeit unconscious, insistence of the patient repetitively to co-construct with another familiar maladaptive relational patterns. Although the patient may subjectively experience himself as an "innocent," passive bystander in yet another relationship gone wrong, relational theory points to the unconscious activity and persistence of the patient in forging new-old relationships.

Psychopathology also is evidenced in disruptions of the normative multiple self. When the developmental relational constituents of a given self-state are too traumatic or too utterly incompatible with other experiences, the capacity of the individual to "stand in the spaces" (Bromberg, 1996) of paradox falters and self-states come to exist in rigidly maintained, dissociative demarcation from one another. The more profoundly incompatible the early developmental relational experiences, the more deeply split the various organizations of a patient's self are likely to be. This view of self can be helpful to supervisors, since it may be within the supervisory space that derivatives of the supervised patient's dissociated self-states first are detected in enactments occurring among the members of the treatment and supervisory dyads.

If both the healthy mind and psychopathological processes are structured by and mediated through relationship, it follows that a relational model of psychoanalytically informed treatment focuses intently on the vicissitudes of the therapeutic relationship. Psychoanalysis, in fact, is viewed as constituted by the unique relationship forged within the analytic space by both analyst and patient.

Analysis of transference and countertransference paradigms is the hallmark of any psychoanalytic treatment, no matter what the theoretical bent of the analyst. Where the clinician's theory does very much come into play, however, is in his understanding of what transference and countertransference *are*, his conceptualizations about the way in which each develops, and his clinical approach to the analysis of these central treatment phenomena. In other words, theory tends to dictate the manner in which analyst and patient subjectively and intersubjectively live out and interpret transference and countertransference manifestations, as well as how they choose to talk about what is being experienced.

Relational theory is placed among two-person models of psychological development and psychoanalytic treatment. Relational theorists hold that it is essentially meaningless to speak about the patient without considering the influence of the analyst on the patient, or to speak about the analyst-at-work as functioning independently from the impact of the patient. Rather, it is a central premise of relational theory that analyst and patient interpenetrate each other's subjectivities from the beginning and, over the course of treatment, create and re-create one another and themselves in ever more accessible and delineated forms. Thus, transference and countertransference paradigms are mutually determined and shaped by each of the two participant observers of the analytic dyad.

This is not to say that relational theorists negate the patient's predilection to enact in the transference vitally important conscious and unconscious relational patterns. On the contrary, as noted earlier, it is a tenet of the relational theory, as it is for all psychoanalytic thought, that patients seek to shape the analytic relationship to conform to their relationally based fantasies and expectations. Thus, they quite literally attempt to transfer into the analytic space the cognitions, affects, self- and other representations, and body experiences associated with their particular relational histories and their internal, relationally organized worlds. To that extent, there is a certain degree of preordination regarding a given patient's approach to her analytic journey. A given patient, however, encounters a given analyst. Relational theory asserts, therefore, that the transference–countertransference matrix fashioned by a particular patient working with a particular analyst will reflect the verbally and nonverbally, consciously and unconsciously, mutually—albeit asymmetrically—negotiated contributions of each and of both together.

In this way, relational psychoanalysis is constructivist (Hoffman, 1991, 1992). Reality and truth are viewed as perspectival; they are constructions mutually derived by and discussed by analyst and patient. This is not to deny the presence of actual stimuli. For instance, an analyst may shift in his chair when a patient is struggling to verbalize for the first time her profound sense of abandonment when her mother remarried. What the patient and the analyst come to understand about the analyst's potentially disruptive movement, however, is something they construct together; they develop a perspective on its meaning for their work together. Ideally, both remain open to a multiplicity of meanings and even when they arrive at a view of what happened between them at that moment in time, they recognize the incompleteness of what they have constructed. The meanings arrived at during an analysis are never exhaustive; they can only be good enough for now. And, of course, there are times when analyst and patient maintain divergent views of something occurring in the patient's life or in the room between them. It is not agreement but, rather, respectful and persistent identification and explication of many possible meanings that constitute relational analysis. An irreconcilable disagreement that honors the subjectivity of each participating observer is a more successful analytic outcome on any given issue than a capitulation of either party to the other's viewpoint when that submission is experienced as inauthentic.

Relational theory accepts that the person of the analyst inevitably influences the development and course of transference and countertransference paradigms. The therapist's own unique tapestry of historical and current relationally mediated experiences, affects, cognitions, somatic states, and multiple organizations of self all are present in the consultation room and engage with those same aspects of the patient's psychic apparatus to co-create a new, unique interpersonal field. What transpires during any analytic journey, therefore, is mutually determined and mutually negotiated by analyst and patient within their admittedly asymmetrical relationship.

Since the analyst is a full partner in the therapeutic relationship, the objectivity of the therapist as an authoritative observer and interpreter of the patient's psychic processes is deprivileged. Rather, the relational approach cites as inevitable the analyst's temporary immersion in enactments of transference and countertransference constellations. It is assumed that, often for protracted periods of time, analyst and patient will live out unsymbolized and uninterpreted relational patterns key to the patient's psychic functioning. At some points, neither party will have the capacity to stand back, to observe, or to make explicit what is occurring on the analytic relational scene. It is the ability of the analyst, in fact, to submit to transference and countertransference enactments and, then, to reclaim an observational stance—to play fully with both participation and observation—that allows treatment to progress.

In this way of working clinically, traditional psychoanalytic concepts such as neutrality and abstinence take on new meaning. Neutrality, for instance, no longer implies maintenance of equidistance from the patient's psychic structures or relational disengagement from his modes of functioning. Rather, in a relational model, analytic neutrality connotes the therapist's ability to keep fluid the relational enactments taking place in the treatment room, to note and bring to the patient's attention the bogging down of transference and countertransference in rigidly endless reenactments of one relational constellation at the expense of all others (Davies and Frawley, 1994). Similarly, abstinence no longer refers to a "blank screen" stance by the analyst. In a relational model, it is deemed inevitable that many symbolic gratifications will occur, particularly as prematurely foreclosed developmental processes are awakened in the patient. Abstinence here refers therefore to the therapist's efforts to maintain openness and malleability within the potential space of the analysis; to attempt to avoid the kind of concretized gratifications that threaten the viability and vitality of the transitional space (Davies and Frawley, 1994). So while it would not be in keeping with the definitions of neutrality and abstinence used in this book actually to take a patient to Disneyland for vacation, many relationalists might consider it quite therapeutic to visit Disneyland with the patient in a shared fantasy, in which *both* analyst and patient embellish a mutually constructed narrative of the trip. In this instance, once-forestalled relational yearnings for play and being special to someone special can flower in the safety and possibility of the analytic space.

It can be inferred from the preceding example that, in a relational model, regression is expected and accepted during analytic treatment. Far from being viewed as resistance or as necessary but wholly pathological phenomena, regressive experiences are viewed as important windows on the internal world of the patient. In fact, they are experiential precipitates of the patient's earlier relational templates that, when lived out with the analyst, eventually can be analyzed, unfrozen from the past, released from their role as propellants of repetitive unfulfilling or even traumatic relational reenactments, and more adaptively configured through the new relationship between analyst and patient. Furthermore, relational theory widens the potential for regression within psychoanalysis by identifying as not only acceptable but also even necessary the analyst's willingness and capacity to permit his own regressive experiences to evolve during his work with a patient. Whether or not the analyst ever chooses to disclose these experiences to the patient—a matter of considerable ongoing controversy, he does allow himself freely and fully to submit to and analyze his own regressive phenomena. Like all aspects of psychoanalysis, regression is conceptualized as a two-person process, mutually regulated by therapist and patient (Aron and Bushra, 1998). It is to be expected, therefore, that during a psychoanalytic encounter, the analyst's somatic states, affects, fantasies, cognitive schemas, use of language, relational strivings, and sense of self often will shift in concordance or complementarity (Racker, 1968) with the patient's own changing states of self. These regressive phenomena in the analyst can help him eventually to elucidate the vicissitudes of the transference–countertransference matrix operating within the treatment and are to be reflected on as potentially valuable postcards from the current imperfectly formulated relational scene.

Some shifts in the transference and countertransference matrix may hearken the arrival into the analytic space of a heretofore dissociated self-state of the patient. In a relational treatment model, the analyst endeavors to invite full participation in and explication of that aspect of the patient's psychic organization and self-structure. The analyst accepts and welcomes elaboration of every organization of the patient's personality, regressive or not, in order to facilitate an optimum capacity to tolerate paradox, with a concurrent decreasing need for defensive dissociation. Here, again, it may be the analyst's awareness of the emergence of various organizations of his own self-structure that cues him to a complementary or concordant shift in the patient. Aron (1996), for instance, suggests that the analyst's capacity to enter into dissociative experiences in himself, in turn, influences the patient's eventual ability to know with some intimacy all of herself.

It is important in evaluating and certainly in applying relational theory to note that mutuality is not synonymous with equality, symmetry, or mutual analysis in the Ferenczian sense. Relational theory does not deny or obscure the real power, expertise, and experience differential inherent and necessary in the therapeutic situation. Patient and analyst have different functions and different requirements (e.g., the patient pays a fee to the analyst); these reflect inescapable and legitimate power gradients (Aron, 1996). In part, the analyst's authority emanates from a socially constructed consensus regarding the training and skills of a professional practicing within a community of professionals and is thus subject to that community's rules of training, ethics, and good practice (Greenberg, 1999). This justification for the power and authority of the practitioner, however, is the point at which most other psychoanalytic models stop. Where the relational model differs from these theories is in its recognition that the analyst's power and authority also are authorized and repeatedly reauthorized through the mutually negotiated ongoingness of the analytic relationship rather than being unilaterally assumed by the therapist. In addition, the analyst's authority is not held to convey unique access to truth regarding the patient's psychological organization, life experiences, or perceptions of the analytic encounter, including perceptions of the analyst. Rather, it is through the analyst's and the patient's increasingly mutual, albeit forever asymmetrical, relational exchange that knowledge about the patient's life gradually is explicated and woven into a narrative that fits what each participant in the analytic dyad, in relationship with the other, has come to accept as true about the patient, her life and psychological organization, the analyst, and their work together. As mentioned earlier, although analyst and patient often will agree on a narrative interpretation of the patient's life and psyche, this model leaves room for difference and disagreement.

With this admittedly schematic presentation of key concepts in relational psychoanalytic theory, we set the stage for our delineation of a relational model of supervision, a model in which supervisor and supervisee participate in and observe their own emerging relationship in a way that provides the supervisory dyad with some analog to the treatment situation.

A MODEL OF RELATIONAL SUPERVISION

Following the typology developed in Chapter 2, we offer our relational model of supervision. We use the three key dimensions along which any supervisory paradigm can be compared with any other. Specifically, we examine (1) the nature of the supervisor's authority, (2) the data considered by the supervisor to be relevant for supervisory processing, and (3) the supervisor's primary mode of participation in the supervisory relationship.

DIMENSION 1. THE NATURE OF THE SUPERVISOR'S AUTHORITY

The legitimacy of the relationally oriented supervisor's power reflects her earned stature in the community, institute, or organization sponsoring the supervision but rests also on the initial and ongoing authorization of the supervisee.

The credentialing of most psychodynamic supervisors, and certainly of supervisors working with psychoanalytic training candidates, implies successful completion or advanced progress in each of the three domains consensually accepted as necessary for psychoanalytic training: didactic classes, supervision, and personal analysis. This credentialing confers upon the supervisor an authority to supervise that is recognized as legitimate by the wider analytic community, institute, or organization to which she belongs. It suggests that the supervisor has the general knowledge, experience, and proficiency to train less advanced members of the psychoanalytic guild. Limiting the source of the supervisor's power and authority to her standing in the psychoanalytic community, however, can lead to a one-person supervisory process in which the supervisor assumes a more omnipotent position than is consistent with a relational perspective.

While the supervisor begins her work with a supervisee with a general authority conferred by her community and/or organization, the power and authority she wields within a specific supervisory relationship is authorized and reauthorized in negotiation with the supervisee. Although the relational supervisor owns and honors her general knowledge and experience, she recognizes that she has no special access to knowledge or truth about her supervisee, the supervised patient, or the psychodynamic work being supervised. Rather, relational supervisory theory asserts that supervisor and supervisee conconstruct, mutually derive, and negotiate meaning about the processes and data of both the therapeutic work being supervised and the supervision. To that extent, supervisor and supervisee share power and authority.

In our delineation of Dimensions 2 and 3—the relevant data of supervision and the supervisor's mode of participation—we emphasize mutuality, negotiation, and distributed power and authority. It is important, therefore, to state clearly that the egalitarianism implied in this paradigm is not synonymous with symmetry any more than the mutuality described in a relational model of clinical work equates to equality between the members of the treatment dyad.

In supervision, as in treatment, there is an inherent, necessary, and helpful asymmetry. As noted earlier, other members of the psychoanalytic community acknowledge the supervisor as having knowledge, experience, and skills that are not yet as fully developed in the supervisee. In addition, the supervisor is paid a fee, often has an evaluative function, and usually prescribes other elements of the supervisory frame, such as where the supervision takes place. At the same time, the supervisory asymmetry often is less pronounced and potentially more temporary than that of a patient–analyst relationship. For instance, supervisors are likely to be more "social" with supervisees than analysts are with patients, sharing plans for an upcoming weekend, recommending a good movie, and, in general, more readily disclosing more personal information than typically is divulged casually to patients. Furthermore, the boundaries between supervisor and supervisee frequently are more flexible than are therapeutic boundaries. They may socialize at professional functions and even become friends, especially after the supervisory relationship has come to an end. Still, during the period of supervisory work, the supervisor has claim to an authority that builds a fundamental and useful inequality into the supervisory relationship.

In conceptualizing the tension existing between power and authority conferred on or assumed by the supervisor and the ongoing authorization of the supervisor's power by the supervisee, we find craftsmanship and the apprenticeship of a craftsperson to be a helpful metaphor. To us, psychoanalysis—and, therefore, psychoanalytic supervision—is neither science nor art but, rather, a craft that combines a number of scientific, theoretical, and technical principles with the inner vision, resources, and artistry of the individual practitioner. To the extent that it can be taught, therefore, it is best taught as craft, with the supervisor taking the role of a more advanced member of the psychoanalytic guild, a practitioner whose own integration of science and art endow her with a breadth and depth of experience as yet not fully available to the supervisee, but who recognizes and respects the uniqueness and value of an individual supervisee's approach to his work.

In this way of thinking about supervision, supervisee and supervisor enter into a relationship through which they participate in the evolution and refinement of the supervisee's uniquely developing craftsmanship. No potter's work, for instance, ever exactly duplicates the artisanship of any other potter. Yet an expert often can detect which elder potters influenced a member of a subsequent generation. Similarly, no analyst practices psychoanalysis exactly as does any other analyst. Yet, each of us probably has had the experience of feeling a perhaps long-past supervisor in the consultation room with us, and we know profoundly at that moment that his or her skills and talents are alive in our own work, kneaded into the very clay of our professional self.

To successfully evoke the greatest potential from his student, the more experienced potter and the learner must together participate in and observe the process of both the apprentice's and the elder potter's work. They share their fantasies and approaches to their work as well as discussing the mutually constructed impact of their collaboration on the apprentice's new work. Likewise, we feel that for the student of psychoanalysis to be able to reach for and freely give voice to his own greatest potential as an analyst, the supervisory process succeeds best as a participation in and observation of analysts—supervisor and supervisee—at different stages of development and at work apart and together. In this way, power and authority are distributed between two professionals, one of whom is acknowledged as having greater general knowledge and experience, but between whom specific knowledge and technique is mutually derived and negotiated.

DIMENSION 2. THE RELEVANT DATA
FOR SUPERVISORY PROCESSING

Dimensions 2 and 3 are highly related. To a great extent, the data on which the supervisor focuses informs his primary mode of relating. For example, a supervisor who considers the patient's psychodynamics to be the most important data is most likely to engage the supervisee in a didactic, or perhaps Socratic way, and is least likely to explore the supervisee's reactions to his patient or to the supervisory process. On the other hand, a supervisor who believes the supervisee's anxieties about the supervised treatment are the most critical content in supervision may engage with the supervisee to clarify, confront, and contain these anxieties. So, while these two dimensions of our supervisory paradigm are considered separately here, it is helpful to keep in mind their inevitable interrelationship.

Relational supervisors consider as pertinent all of the same data held to be important by most psychodynamic supervisors. Like patient-centered supervisors, the relational supervisor works with the supervisee to explicate as fully as possible the depth and breadth of the patient's dynamics. Like the supervisee-centered supervisor, a relationally oriented supervisor is concerned about her supervisee's countertransferences, anxieties, and self-esteem. The relational supervisor, however, sees both the patient's conscious and unconscious expression of his psychodynamics and the supervisee's conscious and unconscious expression of his experiences of the patient, of himself, and of the supervisor as relationally mediated phenomena embedded within the supervisory matrix. This matrix includes, at least, the treatment dyad and the supervisory dyad. Furthermore, the supervisor is assumed to play an actively influential role in co-constructing the relational events taking place in both dyads.

This model of supervision holds that the richest and ultimately most useful supervision takes place when, in addition to more traditional supervisory tasks, the relational vicissitudes of the supervision are examined by both parties as the process unfolds. In this contemporary model of the supervisory encounter, a working assumption is that the more fully and freely supervisor and supervisee represent the intricacies of their own relationship, in particular clarifying centrally related aspects of it to the supervised treatment, the more completely and effectively the supervisee can engage with the patient in identifying and speaking about the relational paradigms operating within the treatment. The medium of supervision is consistent with the message of clinical theory, and the process of supervision parallels the analytic work.

Since the supervisory process is influenced from a number of directions, it is helpful to consider some of the factors that bear upon the supervisory relationship. First are transference and countertransference paradigms that emerge and primarily are reflective of the relationship between a given supervisor and a given supervisee. Included in these may be the evocation of a particular self-state in either supervisor or supervisee that represents the effect of the relational dynamics of this specific supervisory dyad. Second are relational enactments taking place in supervision that bespeak the influence of the supervisee's personal analysis. Other relational processes at play within the supervision may mostly reflect parallels from the supervised treatment. These, too, may be represented by self-state shifts in either the supervisor or the supervisee; in this case, however, they are signals of phenomena primarily emanating from the supervised treatment. Third, supervisor and supervisee may at times enact between them aspects of either or both of their relationships with the organization in which supervision takes place.

Of course, all of these relational factors may be alive in a given supervisory dyad at any one time, adding infinite complexity to the task of mutually constructing a narrative about the supervisory relationship as well as the supervised analytic work. When two or more of these relational processes are simultaneously at work, they exist in dynamic tension, constantly informing, delimiting, and reconfiguring each other like ever-rotating concentric circles. Although they will be considered separately here and in other chapters, it is vital to keep in mind their continuous interpenetration of one another. In this chapter, however, we discuss the transference and countertransference matrices deriving primarily from the relationship unique to a particular supervisory dyad.

It is inevitable that each supervisory relationship will be infused by the development of mutually constructed, co-created transference and countertransference responses that reflect each participant's reactions to the other, mediated by evocation in this relationship of elements of each person's internalized relational world. Here, both transference and countertransference are broadly defined as encompassing each member of the supervisory dyad's full range of relational responses toward the other, and toward himself in relationship with the other. These include, for example, each individual's response to the supervisory frame, a concept roughly analogous to the therapeutic frame and centered, therefore, on issues such as meeting schedules, fee payments, use of tape-recorded treatment sessions during supervision, and so forth. Members of the supervisory dyad also develop relatively conflict-free responses to each other, such as appreciation of one another's sense of humor or use of language. Then, supervisee and supervisor experience conscious and unconscious perceptions of each other's conscious and unconscious, verbal and nonverbal communications, characters, dynamics, and reactions to each other and to the supervised treatment. In addition, the supervisee often brings to the relationship expectations and fantasies derived from exposure to the supervisor's publications, professional presentations and teaching, her reputation in the field, and reports from other supervisees. In turn, the supervisor may begin the supervisory experience with expectations and fantasies about the supervisee based on the latter's performance as a student or what has been said, formally and informally, about the supervisee by others within the program or organization in which the supervision takes place. All of these reactions and responses of supervisee and supervisor to one another, and to themselves in relationship with the other, contribute to the relational matrix within which the supervisory relationship develops.

To set the stage for the members of the supervisory dyad to see the vicissitudes of their own emerging relationship as potentially important grist for the supervisory mill, we think it is helpful if, from the inception of supervision, the supervisor conveys interest in and engagement with the relational process of supervision. Especially since supervisees, particularly less experienced ones, are likely to be unfamiliar with a relational approach to supervision, the supervisor can introduce a relational model such as the one described here to the supervisee, saying something like the following:

> "As we talk about your work with patients this year, we will focus on the relationship that you have with them—on the transference and countertransference matrices you and your patients create together. We certainly will discuss what the patient is bringing to the treatment, and it is also usually very productive to talk about what you are bringing to your work with this or that patient. As we work, we can decide together how deeply into your countertransference reactions we will look, but some focus on them is important in my approach to supervision.
>
> "Similarly, the work we do will occur in the context of the relationship we build during our time together. I hope that, as the year progresses, we can talk about our own relationship and how we perceive ourselves and each other in it, so that we can try to

understand what is happening between us and how it is affecting your development as a therapist. It is also not unusual to find ourselves relating to each other in a way that tells us something about the patient you are presenting. That's called parallel process, and it means that some aspect of the transference and countertransference of the supervised treatment may be acted out in some way between us. So, too, we may find out that something originating in our own relationship parallels into your work with a patient. I have come to believe that the more freely we can speak to each other about our thoughts, feelings, and fantasies about each other, the more fully you will be able to engage in that way with your patients."

Of course, this kind of educational statement would be preceded or followed by a discussion with the supervisee about what he wants or expects from the supervision, as well as the way in which he experiences the supervisor's proposed mode of supervision. Right from the start, then, the supervisor signals that the relational parameters of the supervision are open to some degree of mutual negotiation and construction.

REGRESSION AND DISSOCIATION IN SUPERVISION

In fostering the development of an optimally creative and flexible potential supervisory space, a relational model of supervision accepts as inevitable and therefore welcomes regressive experiences in both the supervisor and supervisee. Despite the fact that current theories of psychoanalytic treatment value mutual regression, the place of regression in supervision has been ignored for the most part. If anything, regression within supervision has been viewed with anxiety, suspicion, and dismay, and has therefore been discouraged. Once again, then, the medium of supervision has not effectively reflected the message of treatment parameters. In our model of supervision, however, it is accepted that both supervisor and supervisee may experience regressive phenomena from time to time during their work together. Like other aspects of their relationship, these regressions may be embedded in transference and countertransference forces specific to their relationship; in processes that parallel in some way the case being supervised;

and/or in aspects of their actual and fantasied relationship with the organization within which the supervision takes place. If supervisor and supervisee are open to regressive experiences that may occur during supervision, and, furthermore, if supervisee and supervisor agree that valuable information about their own relationally mediated work and the supervised therapeutic process may be gleaned from exploration of regressions taking place within the supervisory space, then these become yet another speakable aspect of the supervisory work being conducted.

Dissociative phenomena are a specific category of regressive experiences that potentially hearken the presence of as yet unformulated self-states or transference–countertransference reactions emerging within the supervisory relationship or the supervised analytic relationship. As in treatment, these should be available to the supervisory dyad for elaboration, exploration, and delineation in terms of their meaning. Rather than engaging only with data encoded and expressed through secondary-process verbalizations, the supervisor working within this relational paradigm is open to primary-process data expressed through the dreams, somatic states, fantasies, and regressive and/or dissociative experiences of the supervised patient, the supervisee, and even the supervisor. Often, it is the supervisee who regresses during supervision; equally as often, that regression is embedded in the work with the supervised patient. At other times, the supervisor may regress in a way that offers valuable insights into either the supervised treatment or the supervisory relationship, as the following vignette illustrates.

Carl, a clinical psychology doctoral student with little clinical experience, was in supervision with Jenna, a senior analyst. Despite his inexperience, Carl was remarkably adept in working with the quite primitive material and chaotic histories offered by the three challenging patients assigned to him.

During one supervisory session toward the end of the academic year, Carl presented his work with Stan, a relatively new patient. Stan, a 27-year-old man, sought weekly psychoanalytic psychotherapy because of his difficulty recovering from a broken engagement occurring over a year earlier. The patient reported that he thought constantly about his former fiancée and had even considered stalking her. Depressed, he could not sleep, and was on probation at work because his performance had suffered since the breakup; he had no interest in other women and did not enjoy masturbating anymore—all this despite Stan's conscious feeling that his fiancée had been "beneath" him anyway.

Within weeks of beginning therapy with Carl, Stan's functioning seemed to improve dramatically. He reported feeling more optimistic, said he was sleeping better, left his job for one he described as offering increased financial and career opportunities, and immediately asked a new coworker out on a date. After that first date, Stan told Carl that he had found in his coworker, Samantha, a true soulmate. Stan thought they would probably marry within a year.

The pertinent supervisory session occurred after a therapy session in which Stan described his third date with Samantha, or "Sammy." The evening had ended at Sammy's apartment, where she and Stan began necking and petting. When Stan removed Sammy's blouse, he was surprised to find that she had a great deal of body hair on her shoulders and chest. Then, Sammy suggested that they delay having intercourse because she had some genital scarring, which she wanted to discuss with Stan before he saw it.

Carl talked in supervision about his session with Stan in a calm, straightforward way; when asked, he stated that Stan, too, had been quite reportorial in describing this date, focusing more on his idealization of Sammy and his disappointment in not having intercourse than on the seemingly unusual aspects of Sammy's body. As the supervision proceeded in a somewhat intellectualized way, however, Jenna found herself increasingly on the verge of dissolving into giggles. She also realized that she was reliving in her mind scenes from *The Crying Game*, a movie in which an ostensibly straight man unexpectedly falls in love with a male cross-dresser. The latter does not disclose his biological gender until he undresses in front of his date. The movie raises issues of gender and sexuality in a provocative, daring manner. Jenna, reflecting on her associations and affective response, felt that the giggles might relate to intense anxiety that neither her supervisee nor his patient seemed to be experiencing consciously or at least discussing. She acknowledged to herself that they also represented her own anxiety about discussing this material with a male supervisee.

Despite some apprehension, Jenna decided that her feelings were relevant to the supervisory work. She shared them and her accompanying reflections with Carl, and did, in fact, giggle some while doing so. Looking quite relieved, Carl said he, too, had thought of *The Crying Game* but was embarrassed to bring it up because he worried that Jenna would think it was "too weird." In fact, Carl said he really did not want to know fully his own associations to or feelings about the patient's material because they evoked issues of gender, sexuality, and sexual preference that were disorienting and disturbing to Carl. The supervisee had been raised in a conservative religious community and family in which homosexuality, not to mention transsexualism, was considered an offense against God and thus perverted. Although Carl had rejected that belief system years ago, it was difficult for him to allow to emerge countertransference feelings, fantasies, or body states that threatened his still deeply internalized sense of appropriate sexual and gendered behavior. Jenna responded that issues of gender and sexuality touch deeply primitive experiences in almost everyone, herself included, and that it was not unusual for therapists from all kinds of backgrounds to ward off the affects, fantasies, and experiences of self and other that such material could evoke.

Clearly, there were multiple analytic threads to pursue here relating to Stan's psychodynamics, his internalized relational world, and its expression in his adult relational choices and in the transference to Carl. Similarly, much supervisory attention was paid to Carl's countertransference reactions to Stan and to his anxiety about his supervisor's perceptions of him. Supervisor and supervisee also continued to discuss the dissonance Carl perceived between his consciously held attitudes toward gender and sexuality, and his anxious, inhibited reaction to Stan's material. This was an issue Carl also brought to his personal analysis. Carl and Jenna discussed as well his reactions to her somewhat regressed expression—giggling—of her associations to Stan's material. Pertinent to this discussion of relevant supervisory data, however, is that the supervisory dyad's entry into issues regarding gender and sexuality was precipitated by the supervisor's engagement with, reflection on, and sharing of her own regressive experience, including both her cognitive associations and her affective response.

Very often, clinical material relating to sexuality, aggression, and dependent merger evokes disturbing, primary process and, therefore, too often unspoken reactions in patients, therapists, and supervisors. In this model of supervision, regressive or dissociative experiences concerning this kind of material in any one of the three participant observers in the treatment and supervisory dyads are assumed to hold potential meaning for one or more of the dyads and are therefore considered relevant supervisory data. The supervisor's willingness to make her own regressions or dissociations available for consideration when, after some reflection, she feels they are pertinent to the therapeutic and/or supervisory work models that this material is speakable, containable, analyzable and, therefore, need not be split off.

DIMENSION 3. THE SUPERVISOR'S PRIMARY MODE OF PARTICIPATION

In our relational paradigm, supervision is considered to be an analytic endeavor in and of itself (Rock, 1997). Supervisor and supervisee engage mutually to identify and discuss transference and countertransference patterns, affects, fantasies, defenses, and expectations that further or impede the supervisory process and, thus, the clinical work of the supervisee. Complexity is added to analysis of the supervisory relationship because of its immersion in a complicated matrix of mutually influential relational configurations. At the very least, supervision involves two related dyads: supervisor and supervisee, and supervisee/ therapist and patient. As Fiscalini (1997) says, "The supervisory relationship is a relationship about a relationship about other relationships" (p. 30). Viewed this way, we see that the interpersonal maneuvers and the internalized relational worlds of the three participant observers intersect to define what is seen and heard, and said and done, by whom and about whom. Thus, contemporary constructivist views of the psychoanalytic treatment relationship are expanded here to include supervision. Specifically, in a supervised therapeutic treatment, the patient's narrative—what the patient and therapist come to know about the patient—is co-constructed by the analyst/supervisee, the patient, and the supervisor. When things go well, supervisee and supervisor also may access new strands of their own life narratives.

Herein lie the excitement, the richness, the potential, and the terror of supervision. Through the two dyad's ever more complete delineation of the analytic relationship, mediated in part through increasingly deeper and wider elaboration of the supervisory relationship, *more* becomes possible. The patient comes to know about and be able to speak more about herself, her intrapsychic functioning, and her relational patterns—her affects, cognitions, body states, and fantasies. This occurs, in part, within the context of the supervisee's developing capacity for *more*—more theoretical and technical knowledge, more

insight into his own intrapsychic and interpersonal capacities and limits, more affect, and more confidence in his abilities as an analyst. The
supervisory relationship, in fact, is second only to the therapist's own
analytic relationship in potentiating the supervisee's development as
an analytically informed clinician.

Mutuality and negotiation are the currency of relational supervision. When supervision goes well, it is alive, vibrant and vibrating,
with the cognitive, linguistic, affective, somatic, and relational responses of supervisee and supervisor to the patient and to one another.
It is through the mutual regulation and negotiation of the movement
of supervision that more becomes possible within the potential space
of the supervision and, in turn, within the analytic work of the
supervisee. Even when there is dissonance in one or both of the dyads,
more becomes imaginable, sayable, and playable for the supervisor, supervisor, and patient as co-contributors to the supervisory matrix.

As the process of mutual negotiation and co-narration of the supervisory relationship contributes to the professional development of the
supervisee, the failure of negotiation can divest the supervisory process
of its vitality and creative movement. There are, of course, potentiating
moments of dissonance or relational disjunction that, when named, processed, and worked through, become precipitants to new understandings
and/or heretofore unavailable narrative threads central to the supervised treatment, the supervisory relationship, or both. This is true even
when patient and analyst, or supervisor and supervisee, continue to disagree about the meaning of an event in the patient's life, in the transference and countertransference of the treatment, or in the supervisory relationship. If, however, supervisor and supervisee lose or never establish
the capacity and willingness to mutually negotiate authority; theoretical, technical, and clinical truth; and the ebb and flow of their own particular relationship, the supervision can become mired in the impossible
and the foreclosed. Supervisory impasses can be extremely painful and
can originate in the supervisor, supervisee, or in a terminally non-
facilitative misfit between them. The commitment of each member of
the supervisory dyad to speaking to one another about their experience
of one another in order to negotiate what they "know" about each other,
as well as what they "know" about the supervised patient(s), goes a long
way in preventing such impasses.

A vignette illustrates co-narration between a supervisor and a
supervisee.

Terry was a doctoral clinical psychology supervisee in a psychoanalytically oriented program. About 10 years younger than one of us (Frawley-O'Dea, 1997c), who served as her supervisor, Terry was a particularly skilled and clinically sophisticated woman whose work was a pleasure to supervise. Increasing the satisfaction of the supervisory experience was Terry's openness to exploring her relationship with me as well as the various sources of her responses to patients. I began supervising Terry just a few months after completing my own postdoctoral training and was aware of my own satisfaction at finally having reached full membership in the analytic community. She, in turn, requested me as a supervisor because she perceived me to be a desirable role model for her development as a clinician.

Two months into supervision, when Terry and I were listening to a tape of one of her sessions, we were confronted by the usual static accompanying portable recorders. Spontaneously, I offered to lend to Terry a highly sensitive and powerful microphone I had used as a postdoctoral student and pulled the mike out of my desk, handing it over to her. During the week, I thought about this gesture and realized that, for me, it was more complicated than it might at first appear. In particular, it occurred to me that it represented, among other things, a concretized shedding of my student status. I could turn my microphone over to Terry because I no longer needed it. I was now a grown-up analyst and could lend out the toys of my analytic childhood. As I thought about it, it felt both generative—a passing of the baton and a willingness to share with Terry my powerful analytic instrument—and also somewhat hierarchical, a reminder of who had what status in this supervisory relationship. It seemed to me that there was at least a hint of self-celebration, perhaps at Terry's expense.

In our next session, I asked Terry what her experience had been of the loan of my microphone. She talked about it almost as a transitional object, a way of identifying with me in her own work. Terry further said that she had begun using my office to see her patients, sitting in the chair I used during our supervisory sessions. Terry was conscious only of the generosity and generativity of my loan of the microphone and felt grateful and special to be the recipient of my gesture. As she described her reactions, I saw the admiration on her face and became aware of yet another possible thread to the meaning of my act. A new, fully "hatched" analyst, I may well have hoped for and unconsciously promoted my supervisee's idealization of my hard-won position since, as a matter of fact, I began to realize I idealized it myself!

During the discussion of the microphone, I acknowledged to Terry that there might have been an element of enacted narcissistic self-celebration incorporated in my offer to her. Did she feel any pressure to idealize me or feel so much gratitude toward me, I wondered? She did not think so but was aware of idealizing me and of basking in my compliments regarding her clinical work so far. She went on to say that she rarely formed close mentoring relationships but, when she did, they became extremely important to her and frequently were marked by some degree of initial idealization.

As we began our supervisory year, Terry's yearning to idealize a female role model apparently intersected with my own desire to be idealized as a "real" analyst and was enacted between us around the microphone. While our subsequent discussion did not destroy the ambience of mutual admiration during the supervision, it alerted us and facilitated an openness to the possibility of other experiences of each other that could and did emerge over the year, including feelings of disappointment and annoyance, for example, which also came up and were talked about with some combination of anxiety and comfort. It is my belief that our earlier discussion of the microphone exchange and our delineation of at least some possible meanings attached to it allowed us to speak about other aspects of our relationship as it developed over the year and perhaps prevented it from freezing into a pattern of rigidly maintained mutual idealization.

Yet another aspect of the microphone exchange is notable. Prior to the gesture and our subsequent discussion about it, one focus of my supervision with Terry was to encourage her to be more spontaneous with her patients. She seemed to grasp intellectually that this might be helpful to certain patients, but it was more difficult for her to translate the idea into behavior in the consultation room. In the weeks following our microphone talk, however, I began to hear greater ideational and affective spontaneity on the now much more clearly audible tapes of Terry's sessions. While it is not entirely clear that the microphone incident correlates with this change in Terry's work, I suspect it might. As Rock (1997) points out, within supervision, a "modeling process" (p. 124) occurs. He contends that when supervisor and supervisee engage in constructive dialogue about their relationship, "then the supervisee can do it with his patients. He has the opportunity to gain in courage and confidence that such forthrightness can be therapeutic" (p. 124).

In this vignette, the supervisor discloses openly to the supervisee her subjective experience of the supervisory relationship. Similarly, in the supervision with Jenna and Carl, the supervisor reflected on, then freely shared, her subjective experience of the clinical material and its emergence into the supervisory space. In relational clinical theory, the role of the analyst's self-disclosure remains controversial, although some degree of self-disclosure, especially of the analyst's experience of the clinical encounter, increasingly is accepted as good practice among contemporary, relationally oriented analysts (Aron, 1996; Davies, 1994; Davies and Frawley, 1994; Gerson, 1996; Greenberg, 1995b; Hoffman, 1998; Renik, 1995, 1999).

Within the supervisory relationship, we believe that the supervisor's willingness to share her experience of both the clinical data and the supervisory relationship invites and models collaboration and negotiation. It demystifies the supervisor as an idealized, omniscient, and omnipotent seer and makes available to the supervisee the supervisor's internal analytic processing at work, as best as she understands it, in the moment of the supervisory encounter. Of course, mutuality is maximized when the supervisor offers her self-disclosures as data to be further reflected on and elaborated with the supervisee, and for which new meanings may be discerned through the supervisory dyad's collaboration. In contrast, mutuality is defeated if the supervisor delivers her self-disclosures as "truth," as opposed to data to be considered by both supervisor and supervisee. In addition, a willingness to self-disclose does not imply a requirement to disclose everything the supervisor thinks; there remains room for tact and good judgment in a relational model!

The model of supervision proposed here draws on central principles of relational psychoanalytic treatment to create an analytic supervisory process that is in many ways analogous to the analytic clinical process the supervisee is being asked to learn. The following chapters elaborate more fully key facets of this approach to supervision.

CHAPTER 4

The Supervisor's Knowledge, Power, and Authority, Part I

Mutuality, Asymmetry, and Negotiation

In this chapter, we further elaborate Dimension 1 of our relational model of supervision, that is, the nature of the supervisor's authority. The analyst's authority has been extensively discussed in the contemporary clinical literature, and the issue has recently attracted attention in the supervision literature as well. We explore here the deepening of the supervisory relationship that results when the supervisor views his authority from a postmodern perspective and appreciates the dynamic tensions between mutuality and asymmetry that are inherent in his relationship to his supervisee. The supervisor's willingness to engage in negotiation of conflicts that arise, by honoring both his own and his supervisee's experience, creates a generative supervisory atmosphere. Mutual vulnerability and mutual influence then flourish, and development occurs for members of both dyads.

AUTHORITY IN A POSTMODERN WORLD

The field of psychoanalysis has struggled to define just what kind of authority the analyst can claim within a postmodern world. Mitchell (1997) portrays the dilemma of the analyst who is faced with the difficult task of trying to become an expert on the patient's mind when that mind is viewed as "ambiguous and amenable to multiple interpretations rather than prefigured and distinct" (p. 221). For Mitchell, the analyst "co-creates" the content of the patient's mind from an interactionally embedded position, rather than "uncovering" it from a position of detached objectivity. Analyst and patient jointly arrive at an interpretation of what is going on, but it is in no sense a "best" or a "final" interpretation. Gerson (1996) similarly questions the analyst's claim to authority vis-à-vis technique, expressing skepticism about the motivations underlying the analyst's enduring loyalty to the classical rules of anonymity, neutrality, and abstinence. He attributes that loyalty, at least in part, to the covert use of these technical rules "to maintain hierarchical arrangements of power and privilege in the psychoanalytic situation" (p. 626). As a result of these and other critiques (Aron, 1996; Davies and Frawley, 1994; Greenberg, 1995a, 1999; Hoffman, 1983, 1992, 1996; Mitchell, 1997; B. Pizer, 2000; S. Pizer, 1998; Renik, 1995; Stern, 1997), the authority of the analyst, and by implication, of the supervisor, no longer rests on his role as expert on either the patient's mind or on technique.

Thus, the supervisor working within a contemporary perspective no longer claims a disinterested and objective knowledge of how things "should be done." And the contemporary supervisor can no longer master a coherent body of technical rules and feel that he has learned all that needs to be learned—or what it is necessary to know in order to teach. Once the concept of objectivity is challenged, the analyst's—and the supervisor's—direct experience, tempered by psychoanalytic skepticism and critical reflection, must be considered to be as important a source of expertise as conventional technical wisdom (Hoffman, 1992).

In postmodern psychoanalysis, technique is understood as something that must be freshly rediscovered by a particular therapeutic dyad. Contemporary psychoanalysis recognizes the necessity of adapting technique to the needs of the analyst as well as those of the patient (Hoffman, 1992; Greenberg, 1995a). When the analyst finds herself in a world of meanings rather than absolute truths, she can no longer unilaterally assert "what is true" or "how things should be done" without considering the alternative meanings introduced by the patient. And similarly, the supervisor can no longer unilaterally and authoritatively assert "what is true" or "how things should be done" in the supervised treatment without considering the meanings introduced by both supervisee and patient. Thus, the supervisee, immersed in both the therapeutic and supervisory dyads, finds herself in the position of negotiating with both the patient and the supervisor about how she will work with the patient.

Negotiation has indeed become a nodal concept in the relational literature on analysis (Aron, 1996; Mitchell, 1997; Pizer, 1998) and, consequently, in supervision (Greenberg, 1995a; Leary, 1997). Greenberg, applying the concept to the supervisory relationship, points out that all relationships go through periods of *concordance* and periods of *discordance*. At moments of discordance in supervision—when supervisee and supervisor disagree about the meaning of the patient's or the supervisee's actions, or the nature of the patient's mind, or about the best technical approach to working with him—tensions arise, and negotiation becomes necessary. Continuing to converse through tensions leads to resolution only if the supervisor is willing to take seriously his supervisee's perspective and allow it to influence and modify his own narrative about the nature of the conflict between them, and the best approach to resolving it. The concept of negotiation implies that *both* members of the supervisory dyad have some, although not necessarily equal, authority in deciding what is true and what is best. This more egalitarian attitude is the only one that makes sense within a relational model, which emphasizes the perspectival nature of knowledge.

This shift in power relations dramatically changes how the dyad functions. Take, for example, a vignette offered by Greenberg (1995a) describing his encounter with a supervisee who had apologized to a patient. Greenberg, drawing on his personal view of technique, internalized from his own supervisors, felt strongly that apologies were inappropriate for an analyst to make, and would hamper the analytic process. Yet after unpacking the meanings that he attributed to apologies, he realized that they differed sharply from the meanings attributed to apologies by both members of the supervised clinical dyad. He then decided that he needed to respect the particular meanings that had been constructed by that dyad if he wanted to be of real help to his supervisee. Thus, he concluded that although an apology would indeed have been an unhelpful intervention if *he* had been the analyst, it was, in fact, the only viable intervention for this particular candidate in working with this particular patient.

Greenberg's vignette illustrates how very personal, socially embedded, and therefore nonteachable some aspects of our theory of technique, which we ordinarily take as "simply true," actually are. It also illustrates an important shift that occurs in the supervisory relationship when the supervisor is willing to relinquish a position of authoritative knowledge, and how a process of negotiation can work. In addition, it points up the differences in perspective that can exist between the therapeutic and supervisory dyads, and the tension that this creates for the supervisee as a member of both dyads.

But for every supervisor there are limits to what can—or should be—open to negotiation. Just as the supervisee stands at the intersection of the therapeutic and supervisory dyads, the supervisor stands at the intersection of the supervisory dyad and the values and standards of the broader analytic community (Greenberg, 1999). Any negotiation must somehow take into account the differing interests of all of those parties, and sometimes those interests are not reconcilable. The supervisor has an obligation to stand up for those standards that he finds central to his definition of the work. For Greenberg, for example, although the issue of apologies was negotiable, the issue of the privacy of the analytic consulting room was a core standard that was not open to negotiation with his supervisee. For other supervisors, maintenance of relative analyst anonymity or a certain frequency of analytic sessions may have that same importance. Every supervisor, backed by his identification with the professional community, has core beliefs that he must be willing to uphold or else sacrifice his integrity. The community, with its values and standards—even though those standards are themselves socially constructed and in perpetual flux—thus serves as a stabilizing influence on the supervisory dyad, encouraging the exercise of technical restraint in a postmodern world where technical rules carry diminished authority.

A nonnegotiable disagreement may of course create a rupture in the supervisory relationship. For supervisors who work from a relational model, such ruptures should occur only when the parties truly disagree on core values. Because relational supervisors work within a theory that supports negotiation with different but possibly equally valid alternative positions, they can resolve the majority of disagreements with their supervisees.

The nature of the postmodern supervisor's relationship to knowledge does not lend itself to offering specific technical advice. The supervisor must accept that he can only hope to create retrospectively good-enough understanding of the meaning of what *has already happened* between supervisee and patient (Slavin, 1998). In a sense, then, the relational supervisor is limited to functioning as a kind of "Sunday morning quarterback." He knows that he does not have the capacity to predict or determine exactly how things *should go* in the treatment in the future; that is, he cannot, and should not, attempt to direct the treatment too specifically—what one supervisor described as "treating the patient by remote control." There are just too many variables that the supervisor cannot understand, and too many contingencies that he cannot predict, to make such prospective recommendations advisable. He can tell the supervisee what he has learned from his experience with "situations like this one" but must leave it to the supervisee to apply that knowledge and experience to the case in her own particular way.

Anyone who has supervised knows that it is easier to be clear about what "should be done" with a client when listening to a supervisee's account of a session than when sitting in the session oneself. It is tempting to believe that this ease derives from our superior knowledge and experience, combined with the fact that we are in an "objective" outsider role. But the increased comfort and lucidity that we experience when sitting with supervisees is deceptive and ought not to be taken at face value. It is at least partly an artifact of our position vis-à-vis the supervisee's case material, a position that actually has significant disadvantages as well as advantages. It is true that supervisors do have a certain amount of objectivity as a result of their role as outsider to the therapeutic dyad. But that also means that supervisors are dealing with highly abstracted and diminished data that has been filtered through the psychology of the therapist and is therefore much more difficult to interpret. Supervisors are utterly dependent on the therapist's efforts to condense and communicate not only the verbal to-and-fro of the hour but also all of the nonverbal and affective communication that transpired. From one point of view, the supervisor's pull to think conceptually about clinical material can be understood as a defensive adaptation to the impoverished and contaminated database from which the supervisor operates. It is our way of not feeling stupid when we are confronted with a very difficult and confusing task.

Of course, the supervisor's experience of conceptual clarity may also be reinforced by a supervisee who needs someone who really "knows" what is happening in the clinical encounter. To some extent, the needful trainee–expert supervisor scenario is a necessary one, especially at the beginning of the supervisory relationship, when the degree of anxiety that both participants experience is difficult to bear. Beginners may require concrete and authoritative "answers" until they develop more confidence in their own abilities, and more capacity to think abstractly and complexly about the work (Josephs, 1990). The narcissistic vulnerabilities of the psychotherapy trainee may cause her to idealize her supervisor's understanding as a defense against her own overwhelming feelings of inadequacy in the therapist role (Brightman, 1984–1985). A gradual and nontraumatic process of disillusionment about the nature of the supervisor's knowledge ideally occurs as beginner anxieties decrease and as the supervisor senses that the supervisee can tolerate more ambiguity. What seems crucial is that both participants have some awareness of the arbitrariness and of the defensive components of these roles, and be able to relinquish them when they outlive their usefulness.

Having let go of some of his faith in his conceptual knowledge, the relational supervisor relies on other ways of furthering the supervisee's development and the patient's treatment. He helps the supervisee to examine what already happened in the therapeutic hour, and why she may have found herself feeling and acting as she did. He uses both his accumulated theoretical knowledge—albeit with a more circumspect view of its universal applicability—and his own countertransference experience to do so. He plays with the supervisee to find alternative ways of understanding what has transpired in both the clinical and supervisory relationships. He participates spontaneously, and then steps back to think together with the supervisee about the possible meanings of that participation. Thus, he teaches an approach to participating and reflecting by both precept and example. The contemporary supervisor thus claims a kind of expertise that the supervisor who limits himself to merely being an expert about the patient and about technique does not. The competent relational supervisor is skilled in participating in, observing, and making meaning from the unconscious fantasies, relational themes, affects, and enactments that make up both the supervisory and therapeutic relationships. This is no small challenge, and the supervisor who does this effectively is an expert indeed.

With a diminished sense of the power of his knowledge but an enhanced sense of the value of his experiencing and participation, the supervisor collaborates with a supervisee who has the opportunity to exercise more power in the relationship. As we have already illustrated, in a relational model, the supervisee's point of view *matters* to the supervisor, and when it differs from that of the supervisor, that difference is actively engaged. The supervisee's feelings also matter to the supervisor, because supervisee distress impedes the development of the desired atmosphere of mutual vulnerability and the resulting mutual openness to interpersonal influence. Since the transformative power of the supervisory relationship is understood to reside in this mutual vulnerability and openness to interpersonal influence, the supervisor chooses to encourage the empowerment of his supervisee rather than depending on his power as a supervisor to impress, intimidate, coerce, or instruct (Slavin, 1998).

The relational supervisor thus, paradoxically, has the potential to exercise a degree of interpersonal power and influence that is not available to other supervisors, and that can have profound and far-reaching effects on his supervisees. He seeks to influence his supervisee, with her permission and collaboration, not only cognitively but also affectively. He seeks to engage her true self, not just her professional false self (Eckler-Hart, 1987), by making his own true self available for relating. Deep feelings of attachment and strong identifications sometimes result between supervisor and supervisee, and with them, significant growth and development of the professional—and personal—selves of both participants. The two vignettes from the collaboration of Ella and her supervisor, appearing later in this chapter, illustrate the depth of the relationship that can develop.

MUTUALITY IN THE CONTEXT OF ASYMMETRY

A relational view of the supervisory relationship recognizes a tension between its areas of mutuality and its areas of asymmetry. The supervisor values highly, and tries to optimize, the mutuality of the supervisory relationship. At the same time, he respects and preserves the necessary asymmetries of the relationship. How far can mutuality in supervision go without compromising those necessary asymmetries? What are the risks and anxieties introduced when the supervisor maximizes mutuality, and how can they be addressed?

Contemporary psychoanalysis insists that in the clinical dyad mutuality stand in a dialectical relationship to asymmetry, in order that mutuality not degenerate into merger or an inauthentic sense of equality (Aron, 1996). Mutuality in the context of asymmetry describes our view of the relationship between supervisor and supervisee as well. Like analyst and patient, and parent and child, supervisor and supervisee share a great deal in common, and mutually influence and regulate one another. But just as with parent and child, mutuality in the supervisory relationship exists in the context of important differences in the degree of influence that one participant exerts upon the other, as well as important differences in their roles, functions, and responsibilities. The relational supervisor holds his awareness of these asymmetrical aspects of the relationship in active tension with acknowledging and valuing the qualities that both members of the supervisory pair share in common. He acknowledges that, in many respects, he is more like his supervisee than he is different from her. Both parties participate in regressive experiences. Both participate in enactments and in processing the data thus generated. Both have blind spots and areas of narcissistic vulnerability. Both have particular interests at stake and operate from within particular contexts that affect their participation. Neither party is "objective," since each is embedded in the situation in a particular way.

A supervisor's enhanced appreciation for mutuality creates a sense of safety for the supervisee, and, consequently, an atmosphere conducive to analytic understanding. As one of us (Sarnat) put it elsewhere:

> When the supervisory relationship is viewed as an interaction between two people who are "both children and both neurotics" (Racker, 1957, p. 307), the exploration of supervisee difficulties takes on a very different meaning. Rather than being an indication of the supervisee's failure, or need for more analysis, the presence of such problems becomes ordinary, inevitable, and a subject for analytic curiosity. (J. Sarnat, 1992, p. 396)

When the contemporary supervisor acknowledges the mutuality of the supervisory interaction, he contributes to the pair's ability to work together, increases his interpersonal impact on his student, and models an engaged style of analytic interaction from which the student can learn. But even if acknowledgment of mutuality did not have these positive effects, from a relational perspective, mutuality is a fact of life. Whether the supervisor is willing to make himself vulnerable in the interaction, whether he chooses to see what he has in common with his supervisee, he is unavoidably part of a mutual process that unfolds between himself and his supervisee. Two subjectivities come in to play and together create a unique dyadic process. One of the implications of this view of the supervisory process is that the supervisor's power and authority, like all else, is a co-creation of the dyad (Slavin, 1998). It is not something that the supervisor possesses simply by virtue of his expertise and his authorization by the community. It is, rather, dependent on the authorization of the supervisee, and the supervisee's willingness to be affected.

In some respects, the interplay of mutuality and asymmetry within the supervisory relationship is more complicated and ambiguous than it is within the analytic relationship. For example, in contrast to the therapeutic situation, where patient and therapist can have no legitimate expectation of a posttherapy relationship that will lead to an alteration of the asymmetries of the clinical relationship, today's supervisee often becomes tomorrow's colleague or collaborator. And, of course, a certain amount of extra supervisory contact, during which the two may step out of the roles of supervisor–supervisee and interact on a more level playing field, is common between supervisor and supervisee—when they attend meetings, conferences, and various organizational functions together. In contrast to the therapeutic situation, this extrasupervisory contact, and the multiple role relations that follow from it are generally accepted as a legitimate and nondisruptive aspect of the supervisory relationship[*] and certainly would not be considered intrinsically problematic within our model. The opportunity for a supervisee to interact more informally with her supervisor, and perhaps in a situation where she feels more at ease with her supervisor, can, for some dyads, be a positive experience, diluting a supervisor–supervisee transference–countertransference constellation that might otherwise inhibit openness of expression or ease of collaboration. In other dyads, it can instead increase the level of anxiety. Like everything else in the supervisory relationship, this extrasupervisory contact must be understood in terms of the particular dyad's experience, and be processed within it as needed.

The question arises as to how far this emphasis on mutuality with-

---

[*]See Langs (1994) for a dissenting position on this point.

in the supervisory dyad can profitably go. For instance, the supervisor may worry that by encouraging mutuality in the supervisory relationship, he will lose track of his responsibility as a teacher and allow the supervisory situation to get out of control. He may wonder how he can maintain appropriate focus, and set appropriate limits, on the nature of the relationship. But this is where the supervisor's capacity to hold mutuality in tension with asymmetry comes in: A supervisor will not lose his focus as long as he also sustains his respect for, and ability to stand up for, the necessary asymmetries of the situation.

What are some of the crucial asymmetrical aspects of the supervisory situation? The supervisor carries primary responsibility for defining and maintaining boundaries, for sustaining the dyad's focus on the task, and for sustaining an analytic attitude—or better, for refinding it after repeatedly losing it in the course of the work. He also takes responsibility for assessing the needs of his student and adjusting his approach to meet them. The supervisor stands up for his values and beliefs, taking responsibility for negotiating these when they conflict with those of his supervisee, yet he is prepared for the possibility that some disagreements may not be resolvable. As Stuart Pizer (1999) points out, the supervisor's respect for the instincts of his supervisee cannot displace his exercise of his own best judgment about the treatment process and the patient's welfare. In his view, the responsible supervisor cannot avoid worrying about "dispatching new training recruits into the dense jungle of transference and countertransference enactment, and unconscious communication, without well-maintained regulation equipment" (p. 3), even while holding an awareness of the inhibiting affect of enforcing "standard technique." The supervisor also acknowledges the power that he wields in the relationship as a result of his authorization by the community to teach and to perform evaluative and gatekeeping functions.

One of the most serious consequences of a supervisor's unwillingness to acknowledge the power differential that exists between himself and his supervisee is that he may expect his supervisee to feel safer and freer to express herself than she actually does in the supervisory situation. He may thus leave it to her to bring up difficult subjects that she cannot in fact broach. Most supervisee's feel some degree of intimidation as a result of their supervisor's evaluative authority. A supervisor who does not take this reality seriously and address it directly will hear little from his supervisee about what feels wrong to her in the relationship. But even a supervisor's direct requests for feedback, and his explicit commitment to nonretaliation, will never address all of a supervisee's anxieties. A supervisee also has to test her supervisor, largely unconsciously (Weiss, 1993). Just as we all learn which thoughts and feelings are safe to experience and express with our parents, and which lead to painful disruptions of those crucial relationships, so, too, supervisees are keenly attuned to their supervisors' areas of intolerance and will work hard to avoid them. There is just too much to lose for most trainees to risk challenging such supervisor limitations, and the supervisor does well not to lose sight of this reality.

On the other hand, when a supervisor makes it clear through words and actions that he is prepared to hear about such feelings, engagement deepens, and all members of the supervisory triad grow, as illustrated by the following vignette.

Eight months into a 12-month training year, after a good deal of testing out of her supervisor had already transpired, Ella, the supervisee, started a supervisory session by asking, "Can we process?" She told her supervisor, Cara, that she had felt stung by something that Cara had said during the previous session. They had been talking about how difficult it had been for Ella when Cara had canceled the last supervisory meeting because of an illness in her family. Ella said that as she had been telling Cara how important she was to her, Cara had responded, "Given that I am very important to you—for whatever reason." Ella felt that by throwing in "for whatever reason," Cara had disowned the reality of Ella's attachment to her, distanced herself from her, and made it sound like her involvement with her supervisor was inappropriate and pathological.

Cara tried to remember what her experience had been at that moment. As she reflected, she thought at first that Ella was being overly sensitive. But then she realized that she had felt guilty about canceling the previous session. Cara wondered if her comment had in part been an expression of her need to defend herself by implying, "It's not *my* fault that my absence was so hard for you. You just have an unusually intense attachment to me for some reason that I can't fathom." She told Ella this. Cara also said that she thought that her neglecting to tell Ella about the dates of her summer vacation until the very end of the previous hour (she had been intending to bring it up at the beginning) might have been another expression of her guilt about leaving Ella, and of her difficulty bearing the impact of her coming absence upon Ella. It was surprising and helpful to Ella for Cara to acknowledge that her comment came from her own conflict rather than from an objective and "expert" assessment of the "appropriateness" of Ella's feelings.

However, Cara thought that part of their conflictual interaction came from Ella. She felt that she could now understand better what had previously been a mystery: why Ella's last supervisor, who had seemed otherwise emotionally available, had, according to Ella, totally avoided dealing with their termination. Perhaps it was because her last supervisor had also become anxious about the intensity of Ella's attachment to her. When Cara told Ella that she felt that she could now better understand Ella's experience with her last supervisor, Ella objected to this as well. It felt to Ella as if Cara was again saying that the problem was all in Ella and not at all in herself. Although Cara did not feel that this was true, she did invite Ella to tell her more. Ella said that she had been thinking a lot about the question of whether it is all right to enjoy the fact that a patient—or a supervisee—values one and thinks one is terrific.

This statement of Ella's came as a surprise to Cara. She had been focused on her guilt about disappointing Ella, and had not thought about her response in terms of a conflict about accepting Cara's admiration. Ella said that she felt Cara was unable to let herself enjoy this experience, and wondered if this limitation of Cara's might be contributing to her own difficulty letting herself enjoy a similar experience with her patient, Cindy. Cara acknowledged this possibility and then suggested that causality might point the other way as well, with Ella becoming particularly sensitized to how Cara responded to her expressions of admiration because of anxieties that had been evoked in her by Cindy's expression of such feelings to her.

Ella then presented some process from her last hour with Cindy. As they listened, both observed that Ella had shifted the conversation away from her patient's efforts to tell Ella how helpful she had been to her. Ella had felt that the pleasure she took in hearing this from Cindy was somehow wrong. She said that nowhere in her reading had anyone referred to the legitimacy of the therapist's enjoyment, which left her with the sense that such feelings had no place in the "good" therapist's experience.

Cara told her that this seemed like an important issue for them to discuss, and that she could understand how disquieting her own response to Ella must have been under the circumstances. Cara also referred Ella to papers on idealizing transference–countertransference, and on the therapist's pleasure in the therapeutic process. Here, Ella stopped Cara again, wanting to be clear that she did not view her feelings for Cara as an "idealizing transference." Labeling it that way again felt as if Cara were pathologizing her feelings and distancing from them. The supervisory hour ended on that note.

In this vignette from the latter part of a yearlong supervision, Ella felt free to stand up for herself in a vigorous way, protesting when Cara's responses felt hurtful, and calling Cara on her defensive reactions and avoidances. Having tested out, via tentative expression of her feelings, that Cara was genuinely open to hearing about her experience in the relationship, Ella was now able to express her feelings with confidence, even though they generated anxiety in her supervisor and created conflict between them. Cara managed her anxiety without retaliating and was open to hearing her supervisee out. Ella pushed Cara to renegotiate with her the construction of both the meaning of Ella's intense reactions to interruptions in their relationship and Cara's responses to those reactions. Because Ella felt free to do this, not only did her relationship with her supervisor become more authentic, but aspects of her countertransference to her patient—her conflict about her pleasure in her patient's expression of positive feelings—were also clarified. In addition, Cara learned something about her own anxieties and their possible roots and how these anxieties manifested themselves as resistance to the supervisory work and affected her supervisee.

The feel of this supervisory hour was dramatically different from the earlier months of the supervision, when Ella had taken a much more passive stance, listening to Cara with rapt attention, writing down many of her comments, and anxiously doubting herself while making her supervisor feel like an all-knowing expert. During their 8 months of work, the balance of power between them had realigned as Ella gained confidence in herself and trust in Cara's tolerance for her feelings. She had come to understand the mutual aspects of the supervisory relationship, and to feel free to speak about her supervisor's contributions to it. Even though Ella's persistent confrontation was anxiety provoking for Cara, Ella had learned that her supervisor's conflicts and anxieties could be acknowledged by them both without either losing respect for the other or creating a rupture in their relationship.

We continue with a second vignette from Cara's work with Ella, taken from the very end of their supervisory relationship. This vignette seems to us to demonstrate how mutual empowerment of supervisee and supervisor can result when a supervisor allows her student to teach her, as well as to learn from her; when the supervisor adapts to the supervisee, as well as expecting the supervisee to adapt to her; and when the supervisor allows herself to be vulnerable (Slavin, 1998), while simultaneously maintaining a necessarily asymmetrical role as teacher and role model.

In one of their final meetings, Ella returned to Cara a book that she had borrowed months earlier. She told Cara that she had not been able to finish it, nor had she been able to finish two others that she had checked out from the school library, that she had hoped to finish before the term ended. She said that, at first, she had felt very upset by this, but then she had realized that she did not have to feel pressured to read everything that she wanted to by the end of the year, that she could view her learning as part of an ongoing process, and not one with a rigid deadline. Ella had let Cara know, as illustrated in the previous vignette, that their impending termination was a big deal for her. Her analyst was just about to go on leave as well, so Ella was feeling especially bereft.

After returning the book to Cara, Ella shifted topics, telling Cara, with some distress, that she had left the last supervision feeling bad about herself as a therapist. "You kept telling me what to do with my couple. But your suggestions weren't helpful. They just made me feel incompetent."

Cara compared Ella's feedback to her own memory of the previous session. Ella had presented a couple to Cara for the first time, and Cara had been aware of how little time they had left in the year to talk about Ella's work with them. Cara had had a sense that Ella wanted and needed a great deal of help in learning this different mode of treatment, and Cara had felt anxious about how she could provide enough help with so few supervisory meetings left. Cara then realized that she had been more active than usual in commenting on Ella's work and laying out her own approach to working with couples. Cara could well imagine that the session might have left Ella feeling overwhelmed and inadequate and realized that perhaps she was expressing her own anxiety about their ending through her unusual degree of supervisory activity. As she reflected further upon the session, Cara became more aware of her fears about how Ella would fare without their relationship, and her worry about whether she had given Ella enough during their year of work. Cara decided to tell Ella about her realization, saying, "Maybe I'm dealing with my anxieties about our ending by trying to 'give you all I've got.' " Ella laughed appreciatively as she realized that Cara was acknowledging that she had anxieties, too, and that she had done something to contribute to Ella's.

Then, Cara pointed out that by bringing up a whole new kind of case at the very end of their work, Ella had set up a situation in which they would *both* feel worried about her readiness to end. Ella had, after all, been working with the couple for a number of weeks but had chosen not to present them to Cara until the previous session. Ella agreed that this was so, and they then began to appreciate their mutual resistance to acknowledging their anxieties about ending. Rather than feeling those anxieties, they were enacting a drama in which Ella experienced herself as helpless and dependent, and Cara responded as if that were actually true. Cara also colluded in Ella's unconscious fantasy of a kind of primary dependence upon Cara as a supervisor—that if she did not master this new skill with Cara, it would be a catastrophe, as if there would be no future opportunities for learning after their relationship came to an end.

"Maybe we don't have to finish the whole book before the end of the year and you can keep learning even after our supervision is over," Cara commented, as it suddenly dawned on her that Ella had been unconsciously cueing her about this issue with her comments at the beginning of the session. Cara then complimented Ella on her ability to speak about her feelings and to communicate them in a way that Cara could hear, and that they could both use to create new understanding.

At this moment, something in Ella's manner shifted, and she started to speak in a more self-confident manner. She spent the rest of the session excitedly telling Cara about how well her last couple's session had gone. "Even though your suggestions made me feel anxious, I guess I must have gotten something out of it anyway," she commented, with a grin, as the hour came to an end.

The view of the supervisor's authority developed here, as these vignettes illustrate, supports the empowerment of the supervisee. In the next chapter, we go on to apply our view of the supervisor's knowledge, power, and authority, with its emphasis on mutuality, asymmetry, and negotiation, to a number of specific topics that are central to the supervisory relationship.

CHAPTER 5

The Supervisor's Knowledge, Power, and Authority, Part II

Evaluation, Externality, Sexual Boundaries, and Gender

W e continue our exploration of the supervisor's knowledge, power, and authority by examining several specific topics that are central to structuring the supervisory relationship. Specifically, we look at evaluation, the supervisor as a third party to the clinical dyad, the sexual boundary, and gender, as these areas are illuminated by a contemporary understanding of the nature of the supervisor's authority. We conclude with some reflections on the existential anxieties engendered by our perspective on authority.

EVALUATION IN SUPERVISION

The supervisor has evaluative power, whereas the supervisee is dependent on the positive evaluation of her supervisor. This contrast is perhaps the most significant aspect of the asymmetry of their roles. Even when the supervision takes place outside of a training program that requires formal evaluation, as is the case when licensed professionals voluntarily seek independent consultation, the good opinion of the supervisor matters a great deal to the supervisee. The supervisor can realistically have an influence on the supervisee's reputation within the community, and the supervisee's sometimes unrealistic fantasies about the supervisor's influence in the community can, of course, further augment the supervisee's experience of the supervisor's power.

A supervisor's concerns about competence, oedipal anxieties, aggressive and competitive wishes, or exaggerated fears of his power may lead him to minimize the asymmetry in power that evaluation creates between supervisor and supervisee. It is crucial that the supervisor not disown his power because of his personal discomfort with acknowledging it. The supervisor who does so puts his supervisee at risk, blinding himself to the real possibility of silencing, wounding, intimidating, coercing, or controlling her.

Other supervisors have the opposite difficulty. Rather than feeling uneasy with the asymmetry of the relationship, they feel uncomfortable acknowledging the mutuality of the ongoing working relationship. For some, their discomfort stems from their awareness that at the end of the semester, they will be called upon to evaluate their student, a process that inevitably highlights the asymmetries of the relationship. They dislike the sense of role inconsistency that this shift seems to create. With a difficult student, about whom the supervisor has serious concerns, the transition from the working phase of supervision to the evaluative phase can feel especially jarring. This moment of evaluation can also be experienced by the supervisor as a loyalty conflict: Is the supervisor's loyalty due primarily to the organization requiring the evaluation or to the supervisee? Armed with an understanding of the inevitable tensions between mutuality and asymmetry in the supervisory relationship, the supervisor may feel less caught up in these anxieties, and may make the transition between these two distinct moments in the relationship more gracefully and with a greater sense of role continuity.

The supervisor who anticipates these inevitable tensions can, for example, begin supervision by laying out his approach to evaluation in such a way as to help himself and his student to experience evaluation as an integral part of the work, thus preparing himself and his student for the coming "moment of reckoning" and lessening the shock when it finally arrives. We tend to say something like this to our supervisees at the beginning of supervision:

> "Evaluating you is an important part of my responsibility as your supervisor, and an important aspect of our relationship. I want you to understand from the start how I think about it. I will not

penalize you for showing me your difficulties as long as you are able to consider them and to learn from them. This work is about continually reflecting on one's participation, constantly learning and growing, and I can tell you personally that the process never stops. When it comes to writing evaluations, I tend to feel more positively about supervisees who are taking risks and discussing their areas of ignorance and difficulty than I do about supervisees who provide few opportunities for teaching and learning in supervision.

"At the same time, it is true that if serious and persistent problems in your work arise, I have an obligation to you, to your patients, and to your program to address this. If I have that level of concern about your work, I will not wait for a formal evaluation, and I can promise that you will hear about it before anyone else does. I will work with you to address the problems before I intervene in any other way.

"I also value your feedback to me. It is inevitable that some things I do will not feel useful to you, and it is important to me to know when things don't feel right, so that we can work toward establishing the best possible collaboration. I know that it may be difficult to give me negative feedback because of the power differential between us, but if you offer it to me with care, I will make every effort to reflect upon it and learn from it without retaliating.

"We also both need to keep in mind that our feelings about each other—including our opinions of each other's work—may at times be related to the dynamics of the case we are discussing, and to the dynamics of the organization in which we are embedded, as well as to other conscious and unconscious aspects of our relationship."

Through this kind of statement, we try to communicate to the supervisee both our mindfulness of the asymmetries of the relationship, specifically, our evaluative and gatekeeping functions, and our mindfulness of the areas of mutuality, specifically, our sense of being like our supervisee in our humanity, imperfection, and vulnerability. Supervisees are often relieved to hear that their willingness to be open will earn them respect when we write our evaluations. We find that such an introduction provides a basis for establishing a trusting supervisory relationship and allows us to articulate both for our students and ourselves the necessary complexity of authority relations in supervision.

This introductory statement also asserts that evaluation is not a one-way street. Like all other aspects of interaction, there is inevitably a degree of mutuality in the process. Sometimes that mutuality is formalized, by asking supervisees to evaluate their supervisors in writing, as well as the other way around. We think that such formal evaluative reciprocity is an important aspect of the supervisory relationship and should be standard practice in training programs. However, we should also not forget that the power differential between supervisor and supervisee will inevitably constrain the explicit negative feedback that supervisees will be willing to offer to their supervisors. We find that it works best if both evaluations are discussed within the supervisory pair before being exported to others in the organization, so that each member of the dyad is encouraged to take responsibility for his or her feedback and its impact on the other.

But whether the supervisee's evaluation of her supervisor is given formally in writing to both the supervisor and the sponsoring organization, or informally and verbally to the supervisor, or is expressed only in private conversations with peers and other interested parties, supervisors *do* get evaluated and, inevitably, feel some degree of impact from their students' evaluations. Supervisors value their reputations as much as supervisees do, which gives the supervisee a certain amount of power in the relationship that should not be overlooked.

THE SUPERVISOR AS REPRESENTATIVE OF AN EXTERNAL PERSPECTIVE

Another asymmetry of the supervisory situation results from the fact that supervisor and supervisee each have different outside partners whom they bring with them into their relationship with one another. The supervisee's partner is, of course, her patient, while the supervisor's partner is his community of colleagues, whether formally, if the supervisor works within an organization, or informally, if the supervisor works in private practice. The supervisor, in partnership with his community, introduces an outside perspective on what goes on between the supervisee and her patient.

As we have already suggested, the community serves an important function in both creating and supporting the supervisor's authority. Its presence also keeps alive within supervisor and supervisee an awareness of the existence of an external perspective on what goes on between therapist and patient. Crastnopol (1999), Greenberg (1999), and Muller (1999) have all drawn attention to the importance of this fact, arguing that without the analyst's awareness of the outside world "watching," the analyst could not create an analytic situation. Muller (1999), drawing on the ideas of Lacan (1953), emphasizes the importance of such an outside perspective in maintaining the integrity of the analytic dyad:

> We need the Third* to define our ideals and contain our work. We neglect it at risk because dyads are intrinsically regressive; that is to say, in the deepening dyadic relationship, each of the participants experiences an increasingly all-consuming focus on and by the other as a repetition of the early mother–infant relation. Such regressive propensities, with accompanying narcissistic features, are essential for carrying out the tasks of long-term treatment . . . however the risk is that the dyad will exclude from its field any intervention by a Third, in particular the Third that claims to structure the roles and tasks of each of the participants. (pp. 474–475)

The supervisor represents this third perspective for the supervisee and thus serves the important function of countering the supervisee's potential for merger with her patient. As she sits with her patient, the supervisee, aware that she will soon discuss the work with her supervisor, is thus supported in her dual stance of participation and reflection, of "one foot in" with the patient and "one foot out."

However, our valuing of the supervisor as representative of an external point of view to the therapeutic dyad is counterbalanced by our respect for the wisdom that is intrinsic to the therapeutic dyad itself. With too much intrusion by a too-powerful supervisor, the therapeutic

---

*It is important to note the distinction between Lacan's (1953) use of the term "Third" and Ogden's (1994) use of the term "analytic third." Ogden addressed this terminological confusion. He defined his own "analytic third" as " a product of a unique dialectic generated by/between the separate subjectivities of analyst and analysand within the analytic setting." He contrasted this with the Lacanian "Third," which refers to the father "who intercedes between the mother and infant . . . thus creating the psychological space in which the elaboration of the depressive position and oedipal triangulation occurs" (p. 64).

dyad is in danger of collapsing in the opposite direction, toward a disruption of the sense of protected intimacy, privacy, and freedom necessary for the analytic process to unfold with its own integrity. If a creative tension between the experience within the dyad and an external point of view is not sustained, problems ensue for the supervisee. Technical disagreements can lead to rupture between supervisor and supervisee, unless the distribution of power between them is sufficiently balanced. The following example illustrates how such disagreements may be comfortably held and eventually processed in a supervisory relationship in which power is adequately distributed within the dyad.

Alan, an experienced clinician and analytic candidate, was presenting his analytic work with Dana to Richard. Dana, an unmarried woman in her mid-30s, was working on her seemingly intractable difficulties in allowing herself to fall in love with a man who loved her. She was also, not surprisingly, quite defended against allowing dependent or loving feelings to develop toward her analyst. Richard offered to Alan a series of thoughtful formulations about the dynamics of Dana's inability to love and the transference situation. Although Alan found these ideas interesting, for many months he could not imagine actually stating any of them to Dana. When he was with Dana, Alan found that although he actively struggled to do so, he often had trouble even remembering his supervisor's conceptions.

Richard noted that in the supervisory hours, despite listening respectfully, Alan would often object in one way or another to his comments and seem to lose track of them from supervision to supervision. Richard was frustrated by this fact, but lived with that frustration, and just kept on expressing his view of the case. He developed the idea that Alan's inability to utilize his input had to do with Alan's conflicts around his aggression. He thought that Alan was uncomfortable confronting Dana with interpretations that would cause her anxiety and put him in conflict with her. He mentioned this to Alan, who agreed that this was at least partly true, but nothing shifted as a result of this observation.

This subtle discordance between supervisor and supervisee was only part of what went on between them. The supervisory pair also genuinely liked and respected one another. Richard felt that Alan was working with Dana "well enough," and Alan was finding his supervisor's response "good enough." There were important moments when Richard's emotional steadiness, confidence, and analytic attitude helped

Alan to maintain engagement with Dana in the face of her detachment and subtle devaluing of him, and he was grateful for that supervisory help. Richard likewise appreciated certain elements of Alan's style of working, such as his sensitivity to the psychological surface and to defensive processes. Nonetheless, the discordance created an underlying tension between them that sapped from the supervisory relationship some of its potential pleasure and playfulness.

A year into the supervision, something shifted in both the treatment and the supervision. Suddenly, Alan, struck in a new way with the relevance and usefulness of the ideas that Richard was offering him, found himself applying these ideas in the hours much more actively. Up to this point, Alan had felt helpless to alter the detached, affectless quality of the analytic relationship. Now, suddenly, he felt able to use his supervisor's insights to track Dana's anxieties and defenses against allowing herself to feel need and desire in the transference. He started to use her dream material and other associative material to formulate more complete and vivid interpretations. Dana seemed to be moved by these interpretations. The transference–countertransference intensified, and the treatment deepened.

After a particularly exciting hour, Alan, uncharacteristically, called Richard to tell him about it, and added that Richard's input in the previous supervisory hour had been instrumental in facilitating this productive work. A few days later, he called Richard again to ask advice on managing a frame issue that came up between supervisory hours, and got a prompt response. When, in the next supervisory session, Alan thanked his supervisor for his availability, Richard replied, "It was no problem. I'm into this, too."

At this point, it was obvious to them both that something important had shifted in their working relationship. Richard acknowledged for the first time just how much at odds he had felt with Alan through the previous months. This freed Alan to experience more deeply the disappointment that he, too, had felt in his relationship to his supervisor. Alan said, "I really tried to do it your way. I knew you understood a lot more about psychoanalytic treatment than I did. I asked you to supervise me because I respected your thinking, and liked you. But I *couldn't* do it your way, and stay in tune with Dana. I think we had to do it Dana's way, not just yours or mine."

They now were able to reflect further on the influence that Dana had exercised upon Alan and, indirectly, upon the supervisory relationship. Her reluctance to hear interpretations of the transference–

countertransference had affected both Alan and the supervisory process. Although Richard had not fully understood what was going on between them, he had allowed Alan to have his own relationship with Dana, even while he had continued to offer his different perspective on it.

These reflections led the supervisory dyad to generate a new story about what had been going on throughout this first year of supervision and analysis. Both now felt that Alan's limitations in mobilizing his aggression, although real, were less relevant to Alan's inability to speak his supervisor's interpretations to his patient. Rather, it now seemed, in retrospect, that things had actually unfolded appropriately between therapist and patient. Alan put it this way: "It was as if Dana and I were mother and baby, and you were the father who wanted to push us to separate too soon. All you could see from your position was how Dana should be growing up, analyzing, facing the reality of your formulations, while, from my position, closer to her, I could feel how she wasn't ready to do it yet."

Here, a supervisor showed respect for and sensitivity to his supervisee's work with a patient even while representing vigorously a dissenting point of view. He did not attempt to direct the analysis "by remote control." This supervisor offered his supervisee additional ways of thinking about what was transpiring between him and his patient, but did not disrupt the analytic relationship. The ambience and balance of power within the supervisory dyad allowed the supervisee to resist speaking his supervisor's ideas to his patient when they did not fit comfortably into the relationship, even though those ideas seemed like they *should*, in theory, be useful to the analysis. In part, this was true because Alan was already experienced in the field. But it was also important that this supervisor made space for multiple perspectives and for the evolution of an analytic relationship on its own terms and at its own pace. Members of this supervisory dyad were able to talk about and play with their areas of difference, and to live with them until a moment when it became possible to understand them further and, finally, to resolve them.

THE SEXUAL BOUNDARY IN SUPERVISION

As in psychoanalysis and psychoanalytic psychotherapy, supervision engenders the potential for boundary violations, including violation of the sexual boundary between supervisor and supervisee. Since our approach to supervision, with its emphasis on mutuality, negotiation, and egalitarianism, could be misinterpreted to justify a romantic involvement between supervisor and supervisee as long as it was mutually explored and negotiated, we want to stress the relational and power violation inherent in such an encounter. The supervisor's mode of relating with the supervisee should not include sexual behavior. Sexual behavior, of course, includes any romantic and/or sexual activities as well as actual intercourse.

Although too frequently therapists and patients, including candidates and training analysts (Gabbard, 1999), end up in a sexual relationship (Gabbard and Lester, 1995), the wider therapeutic community is generally unified in its formal disapproval of that outcome. The boundaries of the supervisory relationship, however, are less clear than those of the treatment relationship. Supervisor and supervisee often cross paths at social functions, attend professional meetings together, at times refer patients to one another, and may become friends at some point in time. The supervisor who would never transgress the sexual boundary with a patient, but does have the character structure, life themes, and current stressors that make him vulnerable to sexual acting out (Gabbard and Lester, 1995), may indulge an illusion that to engage sexually with a supervisee is merely to pursue a relationship between equals and is therefore not harmful to the supervisee. The wider professional community may also convey more ambivalence about the sexual transgression of a supervisor than about an analyst who crosses that boundary with a patient. Since the potential legal and career consequences often are *not* as dire for a supervisor who has sex with a supervisee as they can be for a therapist who becomes sexually involved with a patient, the supervisor may experience less prohibition against transgressing sexual boundaries during supervision than during clinical work.

Despite the differences between supervision and treatment, however, supervision remains an asymmetrical relationship with a real power differential, usually including an evaluative dimension. In addition, transference and countertransference are alive and well in supervision, where they need to be reflected upon, discussed, and analyzed to discern their meaning rather than concretely realized. Enactment is not synonymous with acting out. The former values and preserves, while the latter forever destroys symbolization and transformational play.

A high percentage of patients whose therapists engage with them sexually, and/or "fall in love" with them, have histories of early sexual trauma (Gabbard and Lester, 1995; Kluft, 1990). The helping professions also are overrepresented with clinicians who have similar histories (Courtois, 1988; Herman, 1992). All the intense transference and countertransference paradigms that can result in therapists having sex with once sexually abused patients may also come alive in supervision if either or both members of the dyad have been sexually traumatized. The danger in supervision can be that both supervisor and supervisee may fool themselves into believing that supervisory sex and romance are fundamentally different than treatment sex. Instead of recognizing the inherently incestuous nature of sex between supervisor and supervisee, who are, by definition, forbidden sexual objects to one another, both members of the dyad may be more able to split off those implications than they would be as analyst and patient. Gabbard and Lester (1995) make the excellent point that a supervisor who violates the professional boundary required in supervision is not only hurting the trainee but also modeling transgressive behavior for an individual who, through internalization of the supervisor, may then be more careless of boundaries, sexual and otherwise, with patients.

Erotic fantasies and relational strivings that emerge in supervision should be treated analytically, as data from which meaning about the supervised treatment and/or the transference and countertransference of the supervisory dyad may be derived. Do these feelings convey something about the relational matrix of the supervised treatment about which the therapist is currently unaware? Do they represent the sexualization of dependent urges in either the supervisor or the supervisee, or both? Are they suggestive of some avoidance of case material or educational issues by one or both members of the supervisory dyad? Do they signal a transference–countertransference constellation pulling for reenactment of past relational betrayals experienced by supervisor, supervisee, or both? Are they emblematic of rebellion against the training institute or organization sponsoring the supervision? Since secrecy and exclusivity tend to enhance the power of erotic strivings, both supervisor and supervisee are well advised to seek consultation about sexual yearnings or what appears to be romantic love developing toward one another, especially if it seems that an analytic approach is foundering. Since the supervisor is ultimately responsible for maintaining appropriate professional boundaries, it is especially important that he seek consultation in order to contain his desire for the supervisee.

While most analysts insist that once an individual becomes a patient, a sexual relationship with that person is forever taboo—even well after termination, it is not so clear that "once a supervisee, always a supervisee." There is, therefore, the possibility that when supervision ends, a given supervisor and supervisee may explore a romantic relationship for nonpathological and nondestructive reasons. In these probably relatively rare cases, however, it is essential that *before* supervisor and supervisee begin to date or engage with each other sexually, both should seek consultation to explore the many levels of meaning literally embodied in their relationship.

Since the early days of psychoanalysis, sexual acting out of analysts with patients and with each other has marked one way in which the medium of psychoanalytic relationships has deviated sharply from the message (Gabbard, 1999). The model of supervision proposed here insists that supervisors keep the medium consistent with the message when it comes to upholding appropriate professional boundaries in both the treatment and supervisory dyads.

GENDER, POWER, AND AUTHORITY

We cannot leave the matter of power and authority without considering its relevance to issues of gender in supervision. Contemporary gender theory critiques conceptualizations of gender that polarize the nature of the sexes, challenges rigid developmental schemes for gender, and reminds us that conceptions of fixed "gender identity" belie more complex psychoanalytic notions of fantasy, sexuality, and the unconscious (Bassin, 1996; Benjamin, 1995; Butler, 1995; Chodorow, 1992; Dimen, 1991; Elise, 1998; Goldner, 1991; Harris, 1991; May, 1986). In so doing, relational gender theory has done much to rework the simplistic and reified views of gender that characterize earlier psychoanalytic literature. It has also pointed out to supervisor and therapist how destructive such rigid views of gender can be to both supervisees and patients.

This more complex view of gender fits well with a relational construction of the supervisor's authority. Feminist psychoanalysts first pointed out the underlying issues of power and patriarchy represented in the original psychoanalytic view of women and gender. Aron (1996), referencing Phillipson (1993), emphasizes how feminist egalitarianism and the feminist critique of "objective" science have both been instrumental in shaping psychoanalytic relational theory.

In addition, nonpsychoanalytic feminist constructivists have led the way in appreciating that affiliation and involvement are a primary source of the supervisor's influence upon the supervisee. Holloway and Wolleat (1994) note that women have understood this kind of influence process for years. They call this kind of power "power with" rather than "power over" (p. 33), and, like Slavin (1998), they suggest that "power with" creates a distinctly different—and more effective—supervisory ambience. These constructivists also view power as a property of the relationship and not a property of one or the other individual (Hawes, 1992), pointing out that even the lower-power partner can find ways of undermining—or bolstering—the dominant partner's power. Holloway and Wolleat argue that despite the inevitable power inequalities that result from role differences between supervisor and supervisee, the supervisee retains some power by virtue of the fact that her positive feelings for the supervisor are critical for the success of the process. Thus, the supervisor is constrained by consideration of how his actions may affect the affilliative bond between himself and his supervisee.

Nelson and Holloway (1990) conducted empirical research exploring how power and gender interact in supervisory dyads, and from their data, Holloway and Wolleat (1994) draw the following fascinating but disturbing conclusions about the relationship between gender and power in supervision:

> Regardless of gender, supervisors did not support female trainees in expressing their opinions; even when encouraged by supervisors, female trainees were less likely than male trainees to use high-power messages. This study confirms the legitimate power inherent in the role of supervisor regardless of whether a male or female is in the role. Gender role characteristics come to play, however, within the trainee role. . . . That is, supervisors did not encourage female students to break out of a pattern of deference, but did encourage male trainees to increase their use of high-power messages. (pp. 34–35)

Our model's perspective on power—that it is something that should be shared and negotiated, and that it is at least in part co-

constructed between supervisor and supervisee—holds promise for addressing some of the gender-related problems that can limit supervisees. The contemporary supervisor's sensitivity to the typical ways that power and authority play out between men and women is an essential component of actualizing that promise. We live in a world where men often *have* more power than do women, and even when this is not the case, often *feel* themselves to have more power than do women, are *viewed by others* as having more power than do women and, as the above research illustrates, are subtly encouraged to *exercise* more power by those in authority. Given these realities, the supervisor has an active responsibility to attend to and speak about, rather than silently perpetuate, gender-related roles that hold the female supervisee back from experiencing her power (Abramovitz and Abramovitz, 1976; Leighton, 1991; Mendell, 1986, 1993). Any male supervisor who does not actively attend to the subtle ways that women supervisees defer to him, or to the pull he may feel to relate to them as sexual objects, runs the risk of blindly perpetuating traditional gender patterns. Any female supervisor who does not address her male supervisee's anxieties about experiencing the feelings of inadequacy and helplessness that can sometimes underlie anger, or who does not pick up on her female supervisee's avoidance of self-assertion and anger in the supervisory or therapeutic relationships, does her supervisees an equal disservice.

Men's difficulties tolerating women in roles of authority, including their defenses against feelings of powerlessness vis-à-vis the mother (Christiansen, 1996; Leighton, 1991), play a significant role in the perpetuation of traditionally male-dominant authority relations between men and women. Male supervisees should be offered an opportunity to reflect upon the anxieties evoked in them by working with a female supervisor. Female supervisees should likewise get help from their supervisors in empathizing with their male patients' anxieties in working with a female therapist.

Although the supervisor must, of course, assume responsibility for leading the way, both members of the supervisory dyad confront a complex task with respect to gender. First, they need to become aware of their natural inclinations to repeat stereotyped, gendered responses, for example, the supervisor who treats his female student as a sexual object. Second, they both need to acknowledge actual gender differences without assuming that women's styles are pathological because they differ from the (male) norm (Broverman, Vogel, Broverman, Clarkson, and Rosenkranz, 1972; Chodorow, 1978; Gilligan, 1982, cited in Leighton, 1991); for example, women as a group more frequently prioritize care of the other, whereas men as a group more frequently prioritize fairness, and women have more conflicts around autonomy, whereas men have more conflicts around empathic connection. Third, both need to help the supervisee "break from the constraining bonds of their gender socialization" (Holloway and Wolleat, 1994), as, for example, when women inhibit their self-assertion and anger, or when men substitute anger for feelings of helplessness and disappointment. In doing so, a supervisory couple becomes more sensitive to the effects of gender socialization and social pressures of all kinds that limit the supervisee's freedom. This, of course, allows the supervisee to carry a sensitivity to gender issues into her work with patients as well.

The most traditional psychoanalytic view of gender posits a single authoritative narrative of the differences between the sexes. Although most contemporary clinicians appreciate the multiplicity of possible narratives about gender, for many years psychoanalytic clinicians did not, and the issue still arises today, although generally in subtler terms. Two quite unsubtle vignettes, taken from past training experiences, suffice to illustrate the damage than can be done to patients and supervisees by supervisors who nonreflectively treat this traditional narrative about gender as the only truth.

In a weekly case conference attended by all of the staff and trainees at a small agency, a senior male supervisor responded to a presentation of a middle-aged, childless female patient by asserting, "No woman who doesn't have a child can be considered 'fully developed.' " This statement was delivered with a sense of conviction that invited no discussion. Alice, a trainee in the conference, felt intimidated to speak up with her contrary view, for fear of being considered "ignorant about the subtleties of psychoanalytic developmental theory," or "reactively defensive." No faculty of either gender spoke up in the conference to counter this assertion. It was thus allowed to stand, despite the fact that both the patient and the women participants in the case conference were demeaned and stereotyped by it, in a manner that runs counter to the primary values of psychoanalysis and its complex view of fantasy, sexuality, and the unconscious.

Dorothy told her male supervisor, David, about her patient,

Tammy, a childless woman of childbearing age, who had just had a double mastectomy. Dorothy reported that Tammy, expressing a wish to have a baby, had asked her doctor about the medical advisability of this. Tammy's motivation was formulated by David as "trying to make restitution for the lost penis." He said this as if he were informing Dorothy of a scientific fact, as if this were the only legitimate way to understand the meaning of Tammy's expressed wish. Despite liking David as a supervisor, Dorothy never again felt safe to bring a woman patient into their supervision. She was deeply offended by David's comment but felt too intimidated to speak up in protest. Consequently, Dorothy lost out on much that she could have gained from her supervisor, and an important unaddressed area of supervisory disjunction resulted in false self-relating. The patient, of course, lost out, too, when her situation, and her therapist's feelings about it, could not be further explored by her therapist in supervision.

These supervisors did not realize that they were abusing their power "merely" by assuming that traditional psychoanalytic narratives about women were "objectively true." Nor were they aware that they were treating issues that are subject to multiple interpretations as concrete "things" that could be understood in only one way: A woman's decision *not* to have a child does not mean only one thing, any more than does a woman's decision *to have* a child. Haesler (1993), writing about the importance of maintaining "adequate psychoanalytic distance" in supervision, comments on the danger that arises when supervisors, such as those just described, knowingly or unknowingly behave as though their view of the patient is the only valid one. He asserts that psychoanalytic supervision should

> exclude any form of indoctrination, of "teaching" according to criteria of "right or wrong," or of restricting the candidate to just one perspective in viewing the material, rather than allowing the candidate to expand on his points of view and stimulating a reflective attitude which may lead him to justify his opinions with feasible arguments. It is, after all, the feasibility and coherence of conceptualization, and not the theoretical "correctness" of a perception, idea or deduction, that determine "correct" psychoanalytic thinking. (pp. 547–548)

This is certainly true for a supervisor's views about gender, and equally true for a supervisor's views about everything else.

THE EXISTENTIAL ANXIETIES
OF THE CONTEMPORARY SUPERVISOR

The supervisor who functions in a relationship defined by mutual self-disclosure and mutual generation and processing of data makes himself vulnerable, and that vulnerability evokes anxiety. When this vulnerability is combined with the relative lack of certainty that he must tolerate about what he knows and how he knows it, and his understanding of himself as an embedded participant in the process rather than an objective observer of it, the supervisor may feel exposed on many fronts. Slavin (1997) elaborates some of the specific dangers that confront the supervisor and supervisee who take seriously the implications of this new paradigm:

> The danger is that new ideas might undermine the clarity and ways of knowing our theories have provided us. The danger is also of being lost in a complex human relationship without clear guidelines to point the way. Perhaps most of all, the danger is our own intense feelings and of having those feelings exposed and implicated in the treatment relationship. (p. 814)

From a relational perspective, this kind of anxiety is existential in nature: It is inherent in the human condition if that condition is faced squarely and honestly. And it can only be avoided by defensive maneuvers that create other kinds of problems. The supervisor who presents himself as a source of unchallenged expertise and objectivity, or as above psychological conflict and irrational processes, is living a lie. Insisting on such a position creates false self-relating in the supervisory relationship, intimidation of the supervisee, and a pressure for her to conceal the problems and anxieties with which she most needs and wants the supervisor's help. It also creates in the supervisee a sense of mystification that can inhibit her from knowing and expressing her own point of view when it differs from her supervisor's.

The relational supervisor takes comfort in the fact that despite the limitations in his knowledge and understanding, and his inevitable involvement in unconscious enactment, he does not stand alone in his frail humanity, but shares it with all supervisors. He also gains support from a theory that accepts and shows him how to make use of his frailties to advance the supervisory process. Thus, one source of relief for the relational supervisor comes from the holding function of his theory of supervision. Realizing that a theory and a community of peers stand behind him as he stumbles along can make all the difference.

Within a relational model, the supervisor acknowledges his power and authority but views it, and the knowledge upon which it is based, through a postmodern lens. He knows that he, like his supervisee, is a flawed, personally motivated, embedded participant. He also knows that his role carries with it considerable responsibility as well as influence and power that require self-reflection and self-restraint. When supervisors appreciate the mutuality of the supervisory relationship, while simultaneously respecting its necessary asymmetries, they become better teachers, and supervisees become better learners. Empowerment of all members of the supervisory triad results.

CHAPTER 6

Rethinking Regression

In this chapter, we explore Dimension 2, asking what kinds of experiences can become the focus of supervisory attention within a relational model. We argue for the importance of broadening the scope of what may be taken up within the supervisory situation to include what we call "regressive experiences." Supervisory teaching and learning can be greatly enriched by a supervisor who is able to tolerate such experiences and appreciate their value.

Regression, like any concept central to psychoanalysis, has its own history and evolution, starting, of course, with Freud (1900). In his view, it was the analyst's job to help the patient to master and recover from regression, and to do so via the analyst's commitment to abstinence, interpretation, and insight. This attitude grew directly out of Freud's observation of his mentor Breuer's terrifying run-in with an unmanageable erotic transference, in his hypnotic treatment of Anna O (Breuer and Freud, 1893–1895). After this incident, Freud renounced hypnosis in favor of free association, which he felt allowed for a more controlled regressive process. Thus, while maintaining many aspects of the hypnotic situation that promote regression in the psychoanalytic situation—the couch, the quiet, dimly lit room, sitting out of sight of the patient, permission to say anything without fear of judgment, and so on—Freud focused his technique upon abstinence, interpretation, and insight, and renounced the regressive and abreactive potential of the hypnotic method (Stewart, 1992).

Ferenczi held a different attitude toward the technical handling of regression. In contrast to Freud's emphasis on abstinence and insight, Ferenczi saw facilitating the patient's regression back to the original traumatic situation, with the analyst meeting that regression in a new way, as the road to cure. Although his own therapeutic experiments with regression were clinically problematic, analysts who came after him, such as Winnicott (1954) and Balint (1968), developed his ideas with significant therapeutic success.

Just as Ferenczi and his descendants viewed regression as a potentially valuable part of the analytic situation, so, too, do we consider it to be valuable in the supervisory situation. Before elaborating our ideas about supervisory regression, we define our use of the term.

DEFINING REGRESSION

When we speak of regression, we refer to a range of relatively affectively intense and cognitively primitive experiences of supervisee or supervisor. We define this term rather broadly and loosely to capture the kinds of experiences that most supervisees—and supervisors—are not used to acknowledging in the context of their professional roles. These experiences may be understood in terms of regression from secondary process to primary process, regression from reality to fantasy, regression from more complex and mature modes of thinking and feeling to more primitive modes of thinking and feeling, regression from more organized self-states to more primitive self-states, and regression from more mature relational patterns to more infantile modes of relationship. In the way that we use the term, regressive experiences may also include intense affective responses; dreams about the therapy or the supervision, enactments that are generally thought of as evidence of "parallel process," and experiences of altered consciousness, such as dissociative experiences or somatic reactions. We also include among such phenomena the common supervisee experience of disorganization and "de-skilling" (J. Sarnat, 1997), sometimes referred to as "regression in the service of learning," which accompanies many students' efforts to give up old ways of doing things in order to learn something new. Of these phenomena, only parallel process and supervisee reactions to patients (countertransference) are commonly discussed in the supervision literature.

We believe that both supervisee and supervisor regressive experiences are inevitable, and that efforts to exclude these phenomena from the supervisory conversation lead both to an elimination of potentially valuable analytic data and to disruptions in the teaching and learning process. If, on the other hand, such experiences are viewed as part of being human, regardless of one's role, the teaching and learning process deepens, and the supervisory relationship is more likely to weather moments of crisis.

A further comment about our use of the word "regression" is in order, since, despite its roots in the work of Ferenczi, some relational theorists dislike the concept. These analysts take exception to the term "regression" because of its pathologizing connotations and feel that the term unnecessarily concretizes a complex phenomenon. Mitchell (1988), for example, points out the fallacy in assuming that apparent reliving of childhood states in analysis is actually what it seems on the surface. He prefers instead to view "regressive" behavior as a complex construction that combines relational patterns that have evolved within the patient over many years, and current defensive and adaptive strategies.

We agree that the concept requires reinterpretation. For us, like Bromberg (1991), "regression" refers to a progressive and experientially vivid dyadic process in which the subject unconsciously chooses temporarily to delegate to the analyst, supervisor, or supervisory consultant responsibility for observing and containing, in order to loosen his current organization of self so that he may grow. As Bromberg puts it, "The deeper the regression that can be safely allowed by the patient, the richer the experience, and the greater its reverberation on the total organization of the self" (p. 416). The same holds true for the supervisee. The supervisory frame does not invite the same depth of regression as does the analytic frame—in terms of the frequency of meetings, stimulus deprivation when the couch is used, and the degree of ambiguity in the task. Nonetheless, temporary delegation of some of the supervisee's usual adaptive and coping capacities to his supervisor—or that of the supervisor to her consultant—can allow him or her to experience a degree of creative disorganization in the service of growth and development. Regression is thus an important part of the process of structural change for both treatment and supervision.

Therapeutic regression can be "a way of accessing and reconnecting with blocked-off aspects of the imaginal and experiential dimension of life" (Aron and Bushra, 1998, p. 390). The capacity of the subject to move flexibly between more "regressive" and more "mature" modes of experiencing, and to achieve integration, rather than "recovering" from regression once and for all, thus becomes the goal. Similarly, the goal in supervision is to acknowledge regressive experiences and to work toward their integration with reflective processes, in order to deepen and invigorate the supervisory work. The assumption here is that regression will arise in a limited way in supervision and remain indentured to the supervisory task.

From this perspective, a supervisor's availability to work with her supervisee's reveries, dreams, transference reactions, intense affects, or altered states, is essential to fostering the analytic development of her supervisee. Research into the centrality of mutual regulation of states between mother and infant (Beebe and Lachman, 1988; Stern, 1985) has emphasized the importance of the mother's capacity to match the state of her infant, if she is to support the development of the infant's internal object world. Aron and Bushra (1998) similarly emphasize the value of the analyst's attunement to and participation in mutual regulation of states of consciousness with his patient, including regressive states. Just as with mother and infant, and analyst and patient, the supervisor who is able to attune to her supervisee's "altered" consciousness in the supervisory hour contributes to his development, while the supervisor who ignores or avoids such states abandons the supervisee to experiences of disregulation that hamper development.

REGRESSION IN SUPERVISION:
THE CONSERVATIVE POSITION AND ITS LIMITATIONS

Historically, regression in the supervisee has been seen as a disruption to be minimized (Gordon, 1995; Solnit, 1970; Wallerstein, 1981), and regression in the supervisor has been either denied or, if identified, considered to be problematic. The supervisor who views the supervisee's regressive experiences in this way naturally makes no effort to attune to them.

Very real concerns motivate this effort to minimize regressive experiences in supervision. One of the primary rationales for striving to minimize supervisee regression is that if the supervisee is "allowed" to regress, and to develop a transference to the supervisor, then this will create a problem, because the supervisory frame will not allow for its analysis. A supervisor cannot, for example, offer complete confidentiality and is not free to focus exclusively on the personal/developmental needs of the supervisee, since the "real" patient's needs cannot be ignored by the supervisory pair. The assumption is thus made that the transference will inevitably become disruptive, unless the supervisee is induced to "keep it in check," which usually means not talking about it, at least not to the supervisor. And, indeed, this situation does occasionally occur. In the vignette described in Chapter 7, for example, the supervisor needed to terminate the supervision because of Bernie's unmanageable transference to her.

Nonetheless, the main assumption underlying this position deserves rethinking. Transferences are universal and unavoidable in any supervisory situation—indeed, in all relationships—and the question is not whether a transference to the supervisor will be "allowed" to develop, but how fully its existence will be acknowledged, how the supervisee will be made to feel about it, and what use will then be made of it. In this regard, we agree with Etchegoyen's (1991) view of regression in the analytic situation: "The patient *comes* with his regression. . . . What the setting does is to detect it and contain it" (p. 546, in Aron and Bushra, 1998, p. 393). We think this statement applies equally well to the supervisory situation, and we add that not only does the supervisee come with *his* regression, but the supervisor comes with *hers* as well. Preventing supervisee—and supervisor—regressive experience is not an option, and so we do well to acknowledge, contain, and discuss these experiences, rather than casting a blind eye upon them.

Dewald (1987) presents verbatim supervisory transcripts of his extended supervision of an analytic candidate, along with his commentary, offering we believe, a vivid illustration of this point with regard to regression in the supervisee. Dewald gives the impression that he views his supervisory relationship with Dr. Dick as relatively free of conflict, transferences, and other regressive phenomena. However, Dr. Dick paints a different picture in her postscript to the book. She describes her dawning awareness of a powerful split off negative transference to Dewald that surfaced as sudden unaccountable feelings of terror toward him that she could not reconcile with her dominant conscious, positive experience. Once, and only once, early in their work, did Dr. Dick bring these feelings up to Dewald. He heard her out sympathetically but did not encourage her to explore the meaning of her frightening feelings further, and attributed them to an identification with her patient's transference, that is, to a parallel process. Dr. Dick describes her reaction to his comments as follows:

> I was relieved that he responded in such an accepting way; at the same time I felt that he was telling me that this was for me to deal with in my personal analysis. Had I become conscious of the distortion again I would again have forced myself to discuss it with him. I did not. (in Dewald, 1987, p. 459)

We could speculate that Dewald's disinclination to further discuss Dr. Dick's feelings made it difficult for her to risk allowing the experience to become conscious in subsequent supervisory sessions. Dewald's view of supervision neither sensitized him to the importance of such an expression of fear from his supervisee nor allowed him to consider its implications for their work. He may well have mistakenly assumed that he was sparing Dr. Dick unnecessary exposure in the supervisory situation. And so an important area of his supervisee's difficulties, with which she actually would have liked help, was left unaddressed.

Dr. Dick concludes that while this negative transference was present, the supervisory and analytic work were limited for her in a variety of subtle but important ways. For example, she did not feel she could fully accept Dewald's positive evaluation of her work, since she knew she was hiding so much of who she really was from him. Sometimes her supervisor's constructs about the patient also seemed "off" to her, but she had no way to challenge this, or to try to understand what was going on, while her defensive compliance dominated. And, most importantly, she could not fully appreciate her patient's false-self resistances, or help her to resolve them while her own were in place. As is so often the case, this therapist could not provide for her patient what her supervisor could not provide for her. Exploring this "false-self" relatedness in the supervisory relationship, on the other hand, would have facilitated the working through of the parallel form of relatedness in the therapeutic relationship, with the supervisor directly showing the supervisee what was needed, and offering her a new experience that was potentially transformative both professionally and personally.

Stimulated by Dr. Dick's postscript, Dewald accounts for his nonresponse to her transference to him by explaining that she did not

seem more anxious than most candidates, and that he did not therefore feel that her feelings required a response.* However, although
Dewald saw no evidence of "significant interference with the learning
alliance or the candidate's work" (p. 474), Dr. Dick's account indicates that she experienced significant interference of which Dewald
was unaware. When the supervisor feels that it is only necessary to address the supervisee's transference if the supervisee has a clearly articulated or demonstrated problem, issues that need to be addressed sometimes go undetected. The power differential that exists in supervision
causes supervisees to take their cues from their supervisors, and most,
like Dr. Dick, will not pursue issues that they sense their supervisors
are reluctant to discuss. It is our experience that more frequently than
most supervisors realize, the apparent calm and rationality of the analytic therapist-in-training masks primitive terrors, transferences, and
insecurities that are felt to be too dangerous to expose to the supervisor without an active invitation.

This able candidate was eventually able to work through her
transference to Dewald outside of the supervision, and to begin to relate to both Dewald and her patient in more authentic ways. But how
much faster—and farther—the supervisory and analytic processes
might have gone if she and Dewald had been able to talk further about
this transference together!

Ignoring or minimizing the importance of regressive responses
does not make them go away. Instead, exclusion of these experiences
sometimes has the effect of making them more problematic (Epstein,
1997). We agree with Pegeron (1996) that not only does regression
universally occur, but it "may even be necessary in order to achieve
the analytic supervisory goals" (p. 697).

EXPLORING SUPERVISEE REGRESSION

Supervisee regressive reactions can be triggered by the patient, by the
supervisor, or by the learning process itself. We discuss each of these in
turn.

---

*This attitude seems to be widespread. The same pedagogical principle for when to take up
supervisee regressive responses was reiterated by Hirsch (1998), writing not from a classical but
from an interpersonalist perspective: "My proclivity is always to ... deal with supervisor–
supervisee interaction relatively sparingly. What is sparingly? My first inclination it to say, when
I observe a problem in supervision" (pp. 4–5).

The Supervisee's Regressive Responses to the Patient

When the task of supervision includes not only didactic teaching but also exploration of therapist countertransference, the regressive responses of the therapist to the patient naturally move to the fore. The importance of working with therapist countertransference in supervision has been increasingly recognized as the range of patients who are considered psychoanalytically treatable has expanded and models of treatment have changed. Many examples of supervisee regressive responses to patients can be found in that portion of the supervision literature that broadens the definition of the supervisory task beyond the didactic and patient-focused realm (e.g., Brightman, 1984–1985; Eckstein and Wallerstein, 1972; Jarmon, 1990; Newirth, 1990). For example, Robertson and Yack (1993), a supervisor–candidate pair, write about their work with the candidate's dream about her patient. Even without going into the candidate's associations to the dream, its manifest content clearly communicated the candidate's conflict over aggressive feelings toward her patient. By welcoming this dream into their work, this supervisory pair comfortably acknowledge that the candidate is a person with an unconscious, as well as a reflective professional.

Elsewhere, one of us (Frawley-O'Dea, 1997b) offers an example of her own experience of a regressive countertransference reaction to a patient. Frawley-O'Dea had been unable to allow herself to experience fully her reactions to the primitive rage and chaos of the inner world of her patient, Jeff, during sessions with him. With the support of her supervisor, she did so in a supervisory hour, surrendering herself to rising nausea and "rapidly shifting images of Jeff shoving his customer's head into the snow . . . and, then, of disembodied penises, breasts, and heads catapulting through outer space," and the feeling that she was "going to fall off the edge of the world into a never-ending abyss" (p. 16). As a result of experiencing this moment with her supervisor, she was able to progress in her work with Jeff.

The Supervisee's Regressive Responses to the Supervisor

Supervisees also experience frequent regressive reactions to supervisors. The supervisory situation, like the therapeutic situation, echoes the infantile situation in important ways. The supervisee finds himself depending on someone who is generally more experienced, and who is always of higher status, at a moment when he feels anxious and incompetent, and thus in real need. In this asymmetrical situation, the supervisee's needs are prioritized, and he does most of the self-revelation. The supervisor has a great deal more power (both evaluative and interpersonal) than the student. In all of these ways, the supervisory relationship, like any relationship between a learner and a teacher, invites regression in the more dependent member of the dyad.

There are a few examples of supervisee regressive reactions to their supervisors described in the literature. Langs (1984) reports a supervisee's dream that served to bring out aspects of the supervisee's experience of the supervisor that were highly conflictual and might otherwise not have found their way into the supervisory dialogue. Ogden (1997) demonstrates how exploration of his supervisee's subtle negative transference to him, expressed in a supervisee's reverie during an analytic hour with the supervised patient, led to crucial new understanding and enlivening of the analysis.

Bruzzone, Casaula, Jimenez, and Jordan (1985) published one of the few descriptions by candidates of their experiences in psychoanalytic training. Generally, trainees are reluctant to speak openly—much less write—about the degree of anxiety and regression that they experience during the training process. This paper was written only *after* these candidates had graduated. They emphasize the regressive pull that accompanies finding oneself dependent on a supervisor:

> We shared a feeling of having attained a certain maturity which contrasted with our feelings as candidates. . . . Our behavior was more akin to that of a baby who expects everything from an omniscient and idealized being, who at the same time feels totally incapable of thinking for itself. . . . The moment of maximum persecution seems to have coincided with the beginning of individual and group supervisions. . . . Fiercely claustrophobic anxieties made their appearance, as did feelings both of loneliness and incompetence towards our patients. (pp. 411–412)

This description communicates the intensity of regression that we think is typical in the experience of many supervisees, at least at certain moments.

We offer a vignette to illustrate the value of welcoming into supervision the supervisee's regressive responses to her supervisor. After

meeting with Ken in supervision for several weeks, and briefly presenting two other cases, Laurie began to present her work with Linda to
him. Laurie enjoyed Linda, a woman in her late 20s, and felt that she
was being helpful to her. Laurie recounted to Ken a session in which
Linda described a pleasurable fantasy of going to see a warm and nurturing but not terribly skilled hairstylist to get her hair cut. Linda had
interrupted her description of how good this would feel to start criticiz-
ing herself for indulging in the fantasy: The critical side of her insisted
that the haircut that she could get from this woman would not look
"good enough." Laurie felt that the interruption represented the intrusion of Linda's internalized "judgmental mother," who seemed to value
appearances over feelings and needs, and she related this to Linda.
This image of a judging mother who criticized her wishes for simple
closeness and sensual pleasure had recently come up in her transference to Laurie as well.

As Laurie was talking about the session in supervision, she became aware that Ken was beginning to frown. Suddenly, almost without realizing that she was doing it, Laurie heard herself shift to a different stance in talking about her work, and she started expressing
skepticism about her work with Linda, questioning what else might lie
beneath her sense of comfort, understanding, and connection to her.
Ken picked up on her skepticism, and was starting to use it to make an
inference about what was going on in the treatment relationship,
when Laurie was able to grasp that her skeptical tone had more to do
with an anxiety that she was experiencing with *Ken* than it had to do
with her relationship to *Linda*. Laurie decided to stop Ken to tell him
that she now realized that the main reason that she was sounding skeptical was that she felt that *Ken* would call into question the good feelings in the session and assume that something else must "really" be going on underneath.

Ken observed that they seemed at that moment to be repeating
the situation that Linda had represented in her session: two people
happily playing together (Linda and the hairdresser/Linda and Laurie/
Laurie and Ken), interrupted by a judging third (Linda's internalized
mother/Laurie's experience of her supervisor). This seemed vividly
true to Laurie. Suddenly, Laurie became aware of how ambivalent she
felt about presenting this case to Ken, an experience that she had only
been dimly aware of and had pushed aside until that moment. Laurie
was afraid that he would interfere with how she was thinking about

and working with Linda on her own. Laurie wanted to protect their therapeutic relationship from Ken, as though he were a destructive intruder, a view of him that she had not held as she presented other cases to him. The feeling dissipated somewhat as Laurie acknowledged it, and she was left with fuller empathy for the anxieties that Linda was experiencing with her. But Laurie realized how powerfully disturbing the expectation of her supervisor's criticism of her work had been for her. In this instance, the supervisor did not volunteer much about his experience that might further clarify the degree to which Laurie's anxiety may have been a response to his thoughts and feelings. However, his quiet listening and the timing of his frown contributed to the cocreation of this moment—even though he was not in fact aware of judgmental feeling in the way that Laurie imagined.

It is important to appreciate how close this dyad came to *not* making space for Laurie's acute anxiety and intense, although transient, negative experience of her supervisor. Her initial feeling was that her reaction was something shameful that she should try to keep to herself. And once this experience had gripped Laurie, she did not feel free to do anything but try to protect herself from attack, until the experience was acknowledged. A leap of faith and her nascent sense of Ken's trustworthiness allowed her to speak of her regressive experience. Once she did, Laurie found that her sense of her supervisor as a persecutory object quickly abated, allowing the supervisory alliance to be reestablished, and their mutual curiosity and collaborative efforts to understand what was going on to recommence. Had she not felt free to tell him, Laurie would have missed the opportunity to understand from the inside out the specifics of her patient's anxiety. She also would have had to retreat from her supervisor into false-self functioning and to find a way to come to terms with this persecutory experience of him on her own.

The Supervisee's Regressive Responses to the Learning Process

The learning process itself can also set in motion a regressive reaction. For students embarking on clinical training, or interrupting their professional functioning in midcareer to continue their training (R. Sarnat, 1952), it is not unusual to experience some degree of regression in the service of learning or "de-skilling" (Seashore, 1975; Singer,

1982), a sense of incompetence and disorganization that accompanies relinquishing familiar ways of structuring one's experience. The supervisee who is undergoing such anxieties must decide whether it is acceptable to acknowledge to his supervisor the full extent of his internal disturbance, or whether he must pretend that this process is not occurring. Eckler-Hart (1987) interviewed clinical psychology graduate students and concluded that most felt a strong pressure to develop a "false professional self" in order to feel respected by supervisors and the training organization as a whole. The freedom to reveal the full force of their anxieties is a luxury that most supervisees do not feel.

The specific focus of the learning regression and how it is experienced in the supervisory relationship will be a co-creation of the supervisor, the supervisee, and the patient(s) treated. If a single patient is being discussed in the supervision, it is often possible to understand the specific nature of the regression as the mutual creation of these three parties. Even if several cases are being discussed in supervision, the supervisee may find himself focusing for a time on a particular patient who evokes a particular aspect of his issues, and here, too, the nature of the regression may be usefully understood as mutually created by the triad.

The supervisor contributes to the mobilization of a generative learning regression by communicating her understanding of issues that the supervisee, often unconsciously, needs and wants to work on. She clarifies learning problems (Ekstein and Wallerstein, 1972) and points out directions for possible growth, while also considering her own part in co-creating difficulties that arise. When this is done with sensitivity to the supervisee's readiness to learn, and to his narcissistic vulnerability and worries about evaluation, a workable learning regression may ensue. It is a regression that, we would argue, the student chooses— both unconsciously and preconsciously—to bring into the supervisory situation because of the perception that his supervisor will hold the disturbance and not criticize him for it or become overanxious about it. The supervisee pursues an often-unconscious plan (Weiss, 1993), seeking out ways that the supervisor may be available to participate in a relationship that differs in important ways from the supervisee's unresolved internalized object relations, and that will allow him to identify in this regard with the supervisor in his work. And the supervisee often focuses on a patient who is struggling with related problems, and who, consequently, mobilizes these issues in the supervisee, and even sometimes functions for the supervisee as his proxy. Then, as supervisor and supervisee discuss the patient's problem, they communicate simultaneously, unconsciously or preconsciously, about the supervisee's problem.

The following account of a 12-week supervision illustrates what can happen even in a relatively brief period if the supervisee feels free to reveal the full extent of her regression in the service of learning, as well as other regressive reactions. For this student, like many, relinquishing her previous way of working, and trying to master a new approach, left her feeling inadequate and raised enormous anxiety.

Lisa, an intern with very limited experience in psychodynamic psychotherapy, was in supervision with Gloria in a brief treatment training setting. Lisa was also in treatment, but her therapist was not psychoanalytically oriented. Her previous placement had been crisis-intervention oriented, and she had been very good at that work.

At the beginning of their supervision, Gloria explained her approach to supervision and communicated her availability to help her student in whatever way seemed most useful. Lisa expressed an interest in learning to identify and use her countertransference in her therapeutic work. During the first few weeks, however, the supervisory process had a didactic feeling, with Lisa requiring considerable concrete help in getting started with her patients. In this first period, Lisa seemed relatively calm and confident despite her inexperience.

In the sixth week, however, the supervisory ambience suddenly shifted. Lisa arrived looking distraught and told Gloria that she was in distress. Lisa said that she suddenly felt intensely critical of her work. Listening to her therapy tapes, which she had only started to do for this supervision, was excruciating. She had felt competent to help patients in a crisis context, but she realized that she was again a beginner when it came to actually doing psychotherapy. To be specific, Lisa worried that she had gone "too far" in response to her patient Tina's admission to her that she sometimes pushed people away. Lisa had responded by telling Tina that she herself had found it difficult to connect to Lisa in their first session, and then worried that this disclosure might have hurt Tina, since Tina had canceled the following session. Lisa's feelings of destructiveness, failure, and shame were intensified by the fact that she had also just received criticism—about a completely separate issue—from another supervisor.

In discussing these painful feelings, Lisa mentioned that, in her

therapy, she had realized that she was experiencing herself as an omnipotent 2-year-old who can destroy everything. "It makes me think of
the 2-year-old in *Honey, I Blew Up the Kid*," Gloria commented,
thinking what a great metaphor the omnipotent 2-year-old was for the
experience of being an awkward beginning therapist with a sense of
having too much power to affect her clients. Lisa said she thought she
had felt too powerful as a child in her family, and that no one had set
appropriate limits for her. Gloria said that Lisa seemed to feel she was
capable of being terribly destructive, even though part of her knew
that her intervention had been far from catastrophic. Lisa agreed.

But then Lisa turned Gloria's comment, which she had initially
experienced as reassuring, against herself. She started to feel that she
was not being rational when she viewed herself as so powerful and destructive, and was in fact now saying to herself internally, "Lisa, what's
the big deal? You are overreacting!" She told Gloria this and observed
that the response of this internal voice reminded her of how her parents would often respond to her distress—by making her feel emotionally dismissed rather than contained. Now, she added with distress, *she*
did not feel up to the challenge of containing her patient's upset feelings, and it might be years before she could work out this issue in her
therapy. Maybe she was not cut out for this work?

At this point, Gloria, who saw Lisa as a supervisee with great potential, told Lisa that she thought that she was going through a frightening but predictable period of regression in the service of learning.
Gloria said that she herself had gone through something similar, as do
most people who take the risk of learning something new. Lisa's mood
shifted, and she seemed to speak from a position of more compassion
for herself. She agreed that it was only since she had started to understand more about what was going on between her patients and herself
that she had become anxious about whether she was doing a good
enough job—before, she had not held herself to so high a standard.
Lisa said she was learning and did not want to go back, but the experience was destabilizing all the same. Gloria wondered if Lisa's relin-
quishment of her old sense of competence and clarity about her work
had left her especially vulnerable to the emergence of the painful experience of herself as destructive. Gloria also invited Lisa to think
about how this frightening image of herself might relate to Tina's internal object world.

Gloria then pointed out that Lisa seemed to think she should be able to contain her own and Tina's anxieties by herself, which was clearly an unrealistic self-expectation at this stage in her training, and perhaps at any stage. Gloria expressed hope that what they were going through in supervision, although difficult, might help Lisa to feel more able to contain her patients' upsets in the future. Gloria then asked Lisa if she had thought of calling her during this difficult week. Lisa said she had wanted to contact Gloria, but felt that she might be annoyed with her for "overreacting." "Like your parents might have been," Gloria said. Lisa agreed with a laugh. The hour ended with Lisa adding that, in actuality, she had been doing pretty well in her sessions, despite all of the anxiety she had been feeling.

During this supervisory hour, Lisa needed to have a particular affective experience with her supervisor in order to proceed in her work with her patient. Her cognitive learning had outstripped her affective development, and, now, the supervisory dyad was working to help her to "catch up." Although Lisa volunteered something about the family origins of her difficulties, and about what was going on in her therapy, and Gloria allowed herself to associate to that material, they kept themselves focused on the task of helping Lisa develop as a psychotherapist.

But even so, more than just "professional development" was addressed as Gloria explored Lisa's anxiety about being destructive, as well as her worry that she would be seen as "overreacting" if she communicated her distress and her need for help. When Gloria spoke as a kind of mother/supervisor to Lisa, telling her that it was acceptable to want emotional support from her, Gloria was inviting Lisa into a relationship experience that could have significant personal impact upon her. Such poignant moments happen frequently in supervisory relationships that acknowledge the universality of regressive experience. And they happen without particular complication, as long as both supervisor and supervisee engage in a process of mutual regulation as to how far the process will go, and as long as the primacy of the supervisory task is kept clearly in mind by the supervisor.

Lisa's struggles with Tina continued. Soon after the supervision session described, Tina called Lisa between appointments, but Lisa was unavailable. Lisa later tried to call Tina back but did not reach her, and she did not respond further to the message Lisa left for her. Tina did, however, arrive for her next appointment. Unfortunately, Lisa was ill that day and only met with Tina briefly to tell her that she could not see her. Tina seemed to accept this and agreed to return for an appointment the following week. Lisa felt that Tina would come, and she indeed did.

In the next supervisory hour, Lisa described this "reunion" session with Tina, who was absolutely furious with Lisa for abandoning her, and let her know it in no uncertain terms. She told Lisa that she had originally called between sessions because she had been rejected by her lover, and that at the time of the call, she was intensely upset. She told Lisa that she had really needed her, and she emphasized how hard it had been when Lisa was unavailable. Lisa's continuing unavailability the next week because of illness had made matters even worse. Tina told Lisa, "I was starting to trust you and now I know that you are just the same as all the others: not there when something bad happens and I need you." As she recounted the session to Gloria, Lisa described experiencing a new capacity to sit with her patient's strong feelings, despite the anxiety and anger that Tina's accusations evoked in her. Lisa told Gloria that she both understood from inside what Tina was feeling and was moved that Tina could express it to her.

Later in the session with Tina, Lisa told her that she had felt quite concerned when Tina called and knew that something significant must have happened, since it was out of character for Tina to call between sessions. But, Lisa told Tina, the nonresponse to her callback, coming on top of Tina's canceling an appointment, had thrown her off, confusing her about whether Tina wanted or needed anything further from her. Tina seemed moved and said, "I pushed you away, didn't I?" A bit later in the hour, Lisa commented with real sadness, "I wish I had understood better how vulnerable you were making yourself by calling. I would have been more persistent in trying to reach you." At this, Tina started sobbing, and said that she now realized this was the kind of reaction she had longed for from her mother.

After describing this sequence to Gloria, Lisa commented that she thought that her own experience of Gloria's emotional availability when she had been upset had allowed her to be present in a new way for Tina. As Lisa spoke, Gloria reflected silently on the parallels between Lisa's beginning to allow herself to depend more on her supervisor and her newfound ability to allow Tina to experience dependence upon her. Lisa said that she now had a different sense of what it was possible to do in brief treatment, and more specifically, what it was possible for *her* to do.

Lisa had come to supervision wanting to learn to use her countertransference to further the work of treatment. And having set this as a goal of supervision, a series of countertransference regressions did indeed emerge during the 12-week supervisory relationship: her feelings of incompetence as she gave up her old ways of working; her feelings of destructive omnipotence; her submission to a critical parent imago; her feelings of helplessness and despair about containing another's distress; and her defenses against experiencing and expressing her own need for emotional containment. In part, these reactions were triggered by events in her relationship with her patient. In part, they were set in motion by Gloria's challenges to her to learn something new, intensified by the scrutiny of her work via taping and following closely the therapeutic process. But Lisa also exercised a degree of choice, both consciously and unconsciously, when she allowed these experiences to emerge with clarity and intensity in supervision. And because of Lisa's introduction of these experiences into the supervisory relationship, Gloria was able to help her to work through some of her internal obstacles to engaging therapeutically with Tina. As a result, the treatment deepened.

THE SUPERVISOR'S REGRESSION

Examples of supervisor regression are relatively rare in the literature. Infrequent as they are, most of these are presented as resulting from a transient identification with the patient's and/or supervisee's difficulty—a parallel process reverberating upward through the supervisory chain. Less often is the supervisor presented as undergoing regressive processes originating in her own transferences to the supervisee or the supervised patient, or to the organization in which the supervision takes place. A few examples of such reactions do, however, exist in the recent supervision literature, including those offered by Berman (1997), Caligor et al. (1984), Hirsh (1997), Pegeron (1996), Rock (1997), J. Sarnat (1992), Stimmel (1995), and Teitelbaum (1990).

Supervisors need a space in which they may safely acknowledge and process their regressive reactions to supervisees. This work is extremely difficult to do in isolation, no matter how "well analyzed" one may be. Supervisors also have to overcome powerful cultural pressures to feel like competent objective experts in order to acknowledge their transferences and other regressive responses. Supervisor consultation groups—whether peer groups or groups led by a consultant—that provide a context in which it is safe for supervisors to explore their own humanity and limitations, serve an important function. We illustrate with a vignette.

Angela, a supervisor, presented her work with Kim, a foreign-born bilingual man, to a consultant-led group for supervisors. Kim, working with patients for the first time, was having serious difficulty grasping the basics of conducting a treatment relationship. He seemed unable to use himself as an instrument or to process his reactions to patients as a means of understanding them. He tried hard to comply with, and copied in a literal way, technical suggestions offered by Angela, but he did not digest these ideas or use his own judgment about how best to adapt them to particular situations.

Initially, Angela told the group, she had found herself feeling sadistic toward Kim when he made what she saw as serious errors with his patients, wanting to shake him and yell at him, "What do you think you are doing?" But since consulting with Kim's case conference leader at his doctoral program, and discovering that she also had a similar perception of Kim as a dysfunctional student, Angela had begun to accept his limitations, and her sadistic feelings had disappeared. More recently, Angela had felt strongly protective of him and was having fantasies of going out of her way for him in a way that previous supervisors had seemed to fail to do, by actively helping him to find his appropriate place in the field of psychology, which, she acknowledged, might not be that of psychodynamic psychotherapist.

After the group discussed the specific nature of Kim's learning problem (Ekstein and Wallerstein, 1972) and how to address it, Angela asked the group to help her to understand why her feelings toward Kim had shifted so suddenly and extremely. "I felt so sadistic before, and now I feel so strongly protective toward him." When the group's consultant asked what thoughts she had about these two responses, Angela wondered whether they were related to the fact that she grew up in a family with an abusive father and an ineffective, nonprotective mother. The consultant commented that, in those terms, she had shifted in her supervisory role from an identification with the abuser, with her supervisee in the role of victimized child, to an identification with the longed-for protective mother, with her supervisee as the loved and protected child. Angela then was able to realize that her relief after her conversation with Kim's case conference leader resulted from her sense that someone else was available to carry the abuser role, which freed her to be in touch with more positive feelings.

The consultant then wondered whether, despite the comfort that the protective-mother role offered Angela and her relief at having extricated herself from the sadism of the abuser role, there might be problems in her remaining too long in that role. Remaining too long within the enactment might create pressure for the case conference leader to assume the role of abuser in the planned joint meeting with the student, as well as leaving Kim in the role of loved but helpless child, a position that did not support his developing autonomy and self-confidence. In addition, Angela was not free to take into account Kim's patients' needs and the educational standards of the graduate school, if she was wedded to an overprotective stance with him. Angela readily saw this, and, turning reflective, began to consider what her possible next steps with Kim might be.

In response to a particular supervisee, Angela regressed from her usual level of relatedness, in which she could tolerate ambivalent feelings, to a more primitive level of relatedness, which caused her to split her hating/sadistic feelings from her loving/protective feelings. She needed the help of her consultation group in order to gain perspective on her reaction and to become more able to move flexibly among her various feelings. Such supervisor experiences are extremely common but tend to be minimized or even ignored by supervisors who do not have a consultant to help process the experience—be it another supervisor, with whom one exchanges peer consultation, a formal consultant, or a consultation group. Just as patients and supervisees need to feel that they have a containing space in which a regression may safely be revealed and processed, so do supervisors.

EXCERPT FROM A TRANSCRIPT OF A SUPERVISORY SESSION

Finally, in order to demonstrate in finer grain our approach to working with regression in supervision, we offer an extended excerpt from a transcript of a supervisory session in which the therapist, Katherine, is significantly regressed, in response to both a crisis in her own life, and the psychotic transference of her most disturbed patient. The session takes place in the middle of a yearlong supervisory relationship.

Katherine was a well-trained, psychoanalytically oriented mental health professional in her 30s, who had been practicing successfully for more than 10 years. She sought consultation from a supervisor because of both a current life crisis—her husband had died several months earlier—and a concern that her long-term cases were not deepening and progressing as fully as they might. She had some idea that this limitation in her work was related to her discomfort in tolerating her patients' transferences and felt that this supervisor would be able to help her with this issue. Katherine was engaged in her own intensive psychotherapy at the time she entered supervision.

The patient being discussed, Jan, a woman in her 50s, had a traumatic history, including the loss of her mother in childbirth and childhood sexual abuse. This patient had suffered her whole life from depression, superficial cutting, compulsive ideation, and intense anxiety, and had come near to hospitalization at several points. She developed a psychotic transference to Katherine after only a few months of treatment, although she was able to function well enough to maintain herself outside of a hospital. There was an aliveness, an intensity in Jan's feelings for Katherine that, although difficult for Katherine, also seemed to hold the potential for a powerfully transformative therapeutic experience. Jan knew about Katherine's loss through a mutual acquaintance.

The excerpt begins about 10 minutes into the supervisory session. Before the excerpt, Katherine had told her supervisor that she had just run into a friend with whom she had been out of touch, and that she had become upset as she told her friend about her husband's death. She cried as she described the conversation. The supervisor listened sympathetically, accepting this painful recital as a necessary prologue to discussion of case material. After a few minutes, Katherine spontaneously turned to discussing Jan, who had been the focus for several supervisory hours.

KATHERINE: I thought I could talk about Jan. In general, there has been a lot between hours with her lately. I get the square root of actually the amount of what there is between hours—for her—but she wrote me a letter, has called me every Friday.

SUPERVISOR: You see her on what day?

KATHERINE: I see her on Tuesday. Since I spoke with you, I got a letter because she was so brimming over with anger and I guess, in that same week, I must have gotten a letter the next day. I got a call Friday and I had taken the children to the zoo for the day, so I got the message at 5, tried to reach her, and was unsuccessful reaching her all weekend. I felt sort of tormented. I tried her in the evening, I tried her at 5, I tried her at 7, at 10. I tried her in the morning, I tried in the afternoon. And I'd sort of gotten into this thing about how much I should be persisting. I didn't feel . . . it wasn't like the time before, where I felt worried that she might kill herself. I felt more . . . I mean part of the countertransference at that point was that I actually had the sense of calling you to ask you about how much I should—not even if I should be worried—but I felt torn about making contact with her on the weekend, and about being taken up with trying to contact her. There are other times with people when I will be absolutely persistent and I ended up . . . I think I forgot to try again on Sunday night. I felt this combination, this conflict about being remiss, and there is a sort of history now. You know I went away on that vacation and I didn't contact her—you know—until the evening of the following day, which felt like it was the answering service's fault and not my fault. But . . . so it may have something to do with the letter that she had sent me.

SUPERVISOR: The letter?

KATHERINE: She sent me another letter.

SUPERVISOR: In the letter she said what?

KATHERINE: Maybe I should get into the hour before that. But anyway, I guess just one theme or a question for me really is, are things getting worse? What's going on with her? It seems like things are—I got another call from her this past Friday, and she just called, apparently, as she says she's been craving to see me in town, and hasn't. She looks for me everywhere. I know the feelings. There's some—not mirroring—but there's some part of my identification . . . I'll bring that up. So she called me on Friday to see if I was there. And I wasn't. She didn't leave a message. When she came in this time, she said, "Where have your been?" She said, "I looked for you everywhere. Are you gone? Are you out of town? Where are you? It's just so weird. Are you OK?" And then she called me yesterday. Thursday. She was off. So she called me after the day after her appointment. I'd just switched from an answering service to a machine. And so it was actually good. I heard her voice on it. I think it really helped her to hear my voice, but she was near tears on the phone, which is very unusual. She said if I could call, could I? Sometimes it helps to hear my voice. She said, "I am just having a terrible separation anxiety. I feel like it's getting worse. I look for you everywhere and I'm thinking about you. I'm just so worried that. . . . " So we talked about it. I thought that there were a number of things that were probably making her anxious on that day. In addition, yesterday—

SUPERVISOR: This was on the phone?

KATHERINE: This was on the phone. She had asked me in the session before—now we get back into the details of the session—but she just said, "Did you just fall asleep? Did you just go to sleep for a minute?" And you know, I didn't, but I had been waking up very early. I think I looked pretty tired. And she said, "Do you get physical checkups every year?" And I said, "Yeah, I do." So I brought that up in the phone call—

SUPERVISOR: That was in the session—

KATHERINE: Yeah. And I said, you know, that I thought that she was struggling with a lot of feelings about me right now, a lot of different kinds of feelings that were making her feel really scared and confused. Some of it was feeling increasingly more dependent on me, and also that she was not getting to be with me as much as she wanted, that she was feeling also very very angry, but that some scary things had happened lately that made her feel particularly scared of what happened when she got angry. And I think the news that she heard about my life added to her worry. That's why I wondered if she had thought any more about why she had been concerned about, you know, my health. She said, "Well, just when people are going through something like you are going through, sometimes they get sick." And I said, "First of all, you know, I think you . . . was there anything in particular yesterday that made you feel a little worried?" She said no. I said, "I wonder if I didn't look more tired to you. I looked tired to myself. And I am a little tired. And I wonder if maybe you are feeling concerned about that." She said, "Well, I just worry because of your situation." And I said, "You know I'm aware, you know, that people can have physical symptoms in my situation, and I really know how to take care of myself. I do yearly checks and I am extremely responsible about that aspect of it, so you don't need to worry. I am a very healthy person." She goes, "I just can't stand the idea of anything happening to you." And I said, "I think that has to do with some-times you get so angry." And she said, "It's true." And I said, "I don't think anything is going to happen to me. You know very well if something did, it wouldn't be your fault." She said, "But I just couldn't deal with it." I said, "Well, one thing about you, Jan, you know you are a fighter. You've been through a lot. If it were that anything happened, you also have what it takes to get through it. Although, you know, I'm not planning for anything to happen. . ."

SUPERVISOR: OK. It's interesting that you're telling me this transac-tion after what we talked about in the last supervision. It's amazing that it's exactly on the same issue, it seems to me, that we were talking about.

KATHERINE: Right. Which is very much in there. I mean, I'll go through the hours. There is all the stuff of her incredible rage, in one session, and then in another session a just being . . . like this last session, when she said, "Can you just tell me a story?" And "I love the way you dress. I wish I could dress like you." You know, both her love for me and her comfort with me and, you know, her complete rage at me, and then her terror between sessions. And she's very, very depressed. She's on medications. It doesn't appear to be working. She's having terrible sleeping problems. She's not even sleeping.

SUPERVISOR: What kind of medication is she on?

KATHERINE: Currently, I think she's on an antidepressant, I think, and something else—Dalmane. She stopped the Dalmane because she felt too groggy. The antidepressant is helping with . . . she has completely stopped cutting, which is feeling like a relief to her, but she's getting these symptoms, which, I think, you know, are side effects. Terrific arthritis in her hands and arms, and it's really not helping with the depression.

SUPERVISOR: I know that you want to give me more process—

KATHERINE: Uh-huh.

SUPERVISOR: But the vignette that you just described to me, the chunk of interaction, feels like it has something in it already that we can talk about.

KATHERINE: Right. The interesting thing with her . . . I mean I don't have process notes, but I feel like we could take . . . I mean more so than with other people, everything seems in every interaction, I mean it—

SUPERVISOR: It's all there. Right on the surface.

KATHERINE: Right. It's like a miniature egg. Everything is there in every interaction so . . . I think we'll capture whatever it is in other places.

SUPERVISOR: What I am picking up on is that this is another place where she is expressing to you very directly a transference fantasy, and an anxiety, and it's almost delusional in quality. I mean, it's so real to her. And there is a technical issue here.

KATHERINE: A transference.

SUPERVISOR: Her worry that she is going to kill you with her need for you, or drive you away. But here, it seems to be that she is going to kill you off, and I think you are absolutely right. I think you see where the separation anxiety is coming from. It's a kind of vicious cycle.

KATHERINE: Right.

SUPERVISOR: The more she needs you, the more she wants to devour you.

KATHERINE: Right.

SUPERVISOR: And the more she wants to devour you, the more worried she is that you can't withstand it, and you're going to get sick, you're going to—

KATHERINE: Which I haven't, sort of, said that to her. I mean, I wondered, you know, because she says to me . . . this is actually why, I think, the reason I wanted to talk to you about this, which I felt wrong in saying. I don't think that is true, but actually, what you say is more validating of what she's been saying: "It's getting worse. I'm getting worse. It's not getting better." And I said . . . she said, "I feel like I'm going crazy." And I sort of denied it, you know, in this attempt to reassure her that I felt was invalidated.

SUPERVISOR: And then what I think happens with you, which we were beginning to talk about last time, is that when she gets into this place, you get so frightened, and you—

KATHERINE: Did we talk about that? (*Laughs.*)

SUPERVISOR: Well we talked about the fact that—

KATHERINE: I can't remember that part. (*Laughs.*)

SUPERVISOR: What I remember is your commenting that you have trouble letting the transference deepen. That you get into a kind of reassuring mode, and I think that with her, it's backfiring. That with her, what's happening is that you're getting pulled a little bit, as anyone would, into her delusional state, and that you—

KATHERINE: Buy into the fact that she could destroy me.

SUPERVISOR: Right.

KATHERINE: I get—

SUPERVISOR: And you're worrying a little bit with her, as you have to. You can't be close to this lady and not. But when that's happening, it's upsetting and scaring you and—

KATHERINE: This is where my countertransference, I mean, not just to her transference, but I don't imagine, I mean, where I identify with her, and there's a lot of it lately. It's funny. In my own therapy, there are some moments when I'll say, "The way I'm acting right now reminds me of my most disturbed patient, Jan." Oftentimes, I find myself doing like this, like she does. You know, I don't ever imagine that I or somebody will die because of what I do, because of my neediness. But I definitely worry about, I mean, I have the same thing as worrying about wearing somebody out, and then wearing them out.

SUPERVISOR: Wearing somebody out, yeah.

KATHERINE: I've been perseverating on needing to call my therapist this week and I haven't. But it has made me completely anxious, and I have an increased need to do it but an increased worry that if I do it, I'm not . . . so there is that moment of identification.

SUPERVISOR: Yes, yes, and that makes it hard for you to work with her feelings toward you because they feel so—

KATHERINE: And I feel like *I'm* falling apart at times and like, when she says, "Am I falling apart now? Will I? You know, people are murderers. People can go from this to being murderers, and am I?" She talked about—

SUPERVISOR: She says this?

KATHERINE: Yeah, well, she talked this time about how, many years ago, when she saw Dr. F, he had said, "You know, you are obsessive–compulsive." She said that she had very obsessive thoughts about wanting to kill her son, and she said to him, "Do you think I'll do it?" And he said, "I don't know." And she said that was soooo frightening to her. . . . It was terribly upsetting to her. She also . . . felt like he was trying to protect himself.

SUPERVISOR: It's interesting that she recounts that to you, because in that story, he did, if we are to take her literally, exactly what you are doing.

KATHERINE: The opposite.

SUPERVISOR: No! In one way, it's different, but on another level, it's the same thing. He was responding to the content of what she was talking about in a reality way, as opposed to making an interpreta-tion, which would have the effect, I think, of calming her, because it would say, "What you are experiencing is feeling."

KATHERINE: Which would calm her. Calm her.

SUPERVISOR: To be able to make an interpretation instead of to give—

KATHERINE: Would calm her.

SUPERVISOR: —a reality answer. Whether you say, "No, you're not going to kill him," or "I don't know whether you're going to kill him." Either way, you're dealing with her on the level of reality.

KATHERINE: Right.

SUPERVISOR: Which is terrifying, because it means you think that this is about real stuff, real actions as opposed to—

KATHERINE: Do you think I'm wrong in reassuring her? I mean, when she said, "Are you well? Do you get checkups?" Should I not? I mean, was that wrong, doing some of that reality check?

SUPERVISOR: What I'm wondering is if, rather than reassuring her when you respond realistically, it worries her more, because it says, "Oh my God, there is something real here. The issue of my thera-pist's actual health is really the issue here. . . . "

KATHERINE: Right. As opposed to?

SUPERVISOR: Ah. As opposed to saying to her, "You know when you get really involved with somebody and start to really depend on somebody and really need somebody, it is so scary for you, and why wouldn't it be? I mean, my God, you know the first person you really depended upon died as you came into the world and you have blamed yourself for that, and your siblings have blamed you for that, you told me. And you became very very involved with your last therapist. And she ended up abruptly leaving you. You know, I think that the more you begin to realize that, in fact, you love me—you are telling me you love me and you need me—you get terrified that it's going to be too much for me, and if everything isn't perfect in my life, in the way I look, it just feels so real to you that you're doing it to me, you're eating me up. And I can't survive." In other words, the intervention here is to shift from the reality, "Are you sick? Are you tired?" to—

KATHERINE: I follow. I understand.

SUPERVISOR: "—this is your fantasy and this is how you feel."

KATHERINE: "The more you depend, the more you get involved with me, the more you're afraid of how destructive that is."

SUPERVISOR: And in there somewhere is also "The more angry you feel that you can't have me every time you need me, or that I'm with my children and you don't see me on the street any more, the more worried you get." There has got to be a tone of, "Of course you feel this way. It's understandable." There has to be a real acceptance that it's understandable that she would have those wishes, she would have those hates, that envy, and that she would be very frightened by it. A kind of calm, matter-of-fact accepting of this whole fantasy she's living in.

KATHERINE: Uh-huh.

SUPERVISOR: What this does, it creates a potential space, a place for playing, a place for fantasy, and it breaks into this state she is in, where it's all real, its all true. These events are happening.

The supervisor began the session by meeting Katherine's regression, accepting both her need to cry and her disorganization. It is noteworthy that despite the fact that Katherine was an intelligent and well-trained professional, in her current state, she was hard to follow during the first part of the hour. All of the supervisor's interventions in the first three pages were efforts to orient himself to the material, since he, too, immediately felt confused. The supervisor wondered about Katherine's degree of disorganization but thought that he knew her well enough to trust that she was able to function in her professional role, and that the regression could be contained and processed within the supervision. The questions that arose for the supervisor in this first part of the session were, therefore, what did this regression mean in terms of the case, and what was Katherine needing from him in order to work more effectively? The supervisor held these questions in mind as he continued to listen and to try to make sense of what Katherine was telling him.

Then, the supervisor began to intervene more actively, trying to draw Katherine's attention to an aspect of how she was engaging with her patient that reminded him of what they had discussed in the previous supervisory session. He did not get much chance to spell out his understanding of the continuities, since Katherine shifted the focus away from a discussion of her own issues, back to the patient's issues. The supervisor backed off for a moment, asking for clarification about the medication that Katherine stated "is not working." This seemed easier for Katherine to discuss than ways in which her own participation "was not working." Here, again, the supervisor adapted to Katherine's needs and exercised tact.

But in the next sequence, the supervisor tried more insistently to bring Katherine's attention to the transference–countertransference issue with which he felt Katherine and her patient were struggling. He began by describing Jan's "worry that she is going to kill you with her need for you . . . the more she wants to devour you, the more worried she is that you can't withstand it and you're going to get sick." This dynamic formulation, which still emphasized the patient's anxieties rather than Katherine's, seemed to free Katherine to become aware of the anxiety that had been evoked in her by Jan's fear that she was getting worse, and was "going crazy," and to realize that she needed help with this anxiety.

This gave the supervisor the opportunity to return to what he had tried to say earlier in the session, which Katherine had not then been able to hear. He clarified Katherine's anxious reaction to Jan's regressive transference. Katherine's discomfort when the supervisor focused on her anxiety was apparent, although she was able to consider it and acknowledge her inability to remember the previous discussion with nervous laughter this time, rather than avoiding it with a change of subject. The supervisor persisted, focusing on Katherine' defensive use of reassurance to manage Jan's anxiety. Although this was a difficult area for Katherine to reflect upon, it was an area with which she had explicitly asked for help. (SUPERVISOR: "What I remember is your commenting that you have trouble letting the transference deepen.") This allowed him to feel that he had permission to push a bit. He then empathized with, and normalized, an aspect of Katherine's regressive reaction—how Katherine naturally felt pulled into Jan's delusions, which allowed Katherine to observe about herself that she "buy[s] into the fact that she could destroy me." This ability to step back from and reflect upon the experience of mutual regression between Jan and herself represented a step forward for Katherine.

This seemed to be a turning point in the supervisory hour. Katherine went on to explore her regression not only as a response to Jan's transference, but also as something that she felt vulnerable to within herself: "In my own therapy there are some moments when I'll say, 'The way I'm acting now reminds me of my most disturbed patient'. . . . You know, I don't ever imagine that I or somebody'll die because of what I do, because of my neediness. But . . . I have the same thing as worrying about wearing somebody out." After Katherine put this into words, she was able to use her supervisor's help in processing her overidentification with her patient, which had been unconsciously expressed earlier in the hour ("And I said . . . she said, "I feel like I'm going crazy.' ").

We can wonder if the crying and disorganization in the first part of the supervisory session may have been, in part, an expression of Katherine's unconscious identification with her patient, a parallel regressive process unconsciously intended to get the supervisor to do for Katherine what she was having trouble doing for Jan. In any case, the supervisor's calm acceptance, adaptation, and understanding showed Katherine what kind of response is most useful at such moments and offered her a different object for identification. The supervisor's mode of participation was thus consistent with the content he was trying to communicate: He contained Katherine's regression as he tried to teach her about containing her patient. Otherwise put, Katherine may have been testing whether her supervisor would be pulled into Katherine's worries about her problems, as she found herself pulled into Jan's worries about herself. When the supervisor was not, Katherine responded by organizing herself and became more insightful about what was going on between her patient and herself.

The session then proceeded with more specific teaching about how to shift from joining in with the patient's concrete mode of generating experience to creating a sense of potential space in the interaction via interpretation. The hope would be that this didactic portion of the session was experienced by Katherine as not only intellectual teaching but also the offer of a kind of platform on which to stand to pull herself out of the regressive swamp in which she was floundering.

This excerpt raises many questions about how far a supervisor may appropriately and profitably go in addressing the anxieties and regressive experiences of his supervisee. In the next chapter, we explore these questions in some depth.

Regressive experiences in the supervisory encounter are frequent rather than unusual events. They enliven the supervisory situation and may become a rich source of information about the supervisory and therapeutic processes. Such moments in supervision can provide an opportunity for the supervisor to demonstrate to the supervisee how regressive phenomena may be processed and understood. Such experiences may also provide an opportunity for the supervisor to learn more about herself and to refine her supervisory functioning. A contemporary view of the supervisory situation supports the creation of a space where regressive phenomena in both supervisee and supervisor may be acknowledged and processed in the service of mutual understanding and the development of the supervisee's analytic self.

CHAPTER 7

The Teach/Treat Issue

Since the early days of psychoanalysis, delineation of an appropriate approach to teaching and "treating" in psychoanalytic training, included in Dimension 3 of our model, has evoked much controversy and debate. Whatever positions analysts took on this topic over the years tended to be strongly held, suggesting that the teach/treat issue generates powerful affects and anxieties. In fact, the teach/treat question probably elicits more doubt and anxiety in supervisors and supervisees than any other aspect of the supervisory relationship.

THE NAYSAYERS: "TREATING" DOES NOT MIX WITH TEACHING

Many analysts argue that supervision should not become a venue for discussion of the supervisee's personality issues (Arlow, 1963; Dewald, 1987; Frijling-Schreuder, 1970; Haesler, 1993; Hirsch, 1997, 1998; Isakower, 1957; Jacobs et al., 1995; Lebovici, 1970; Levenson, 1984; Searles, 1962; Solnit, 1970). These analysts emphasize the overarching, even exclusive, purpose of supervision as facilitating the growth of the supervisee as a professional by focusing on the patient's psychology and on technique. Arlow (1963), at the most conservative end of this school of thought, asserts that, except in very unusual cases, the supervisor should not even comment on what he sees as countertransference difficulties in the therapist/supervisee. Other analysts recognize that discussion of a supervisee's countertransference reactions to a patient might shed light on important facets of the supervised treatment but warn that such explorations must be extremely circumscribed.

Analysts who consider didactic teaching to be the main function of supervision concomitantly hold that the supervisee's personal growth is mostly the purview of her therapy or psychoanalysis. To these analysts, discussion of the supervisee's character structure, dynamic conflicts, or internalized relational world should take place primarily within her own treatment. In addition to this clear emphasis on didactic teaching, the time-limited nature of supervision and its evaluative function are seen as constraints on the supervisory dyad's capacity for productively examining any more than the surface of the supervisee's countertransference, conflicts, or relational dynamics. Furthermore, supervisees are viewed as particularly vulnerable to humiliation by a supervisor-turned-analyst who intrusively treads on the supervisee's psychological functioning.

TO TEACH OR TO TREAT: CONTEMPORARY PERSPECTIVES

As contemporary two-person models of supervision developed, however, analysts ventured to suggest that a rigidly impenetrable boundary between teaching and "treating" in supervision is neither desirable nor truly achievable (Doehrman, 1976; Fosshage, 1997; Frawley-O'Dea, 1997b, 1998; Harris and Ragen, 1995; Issacharoff, 1984; Lesser, 1984; Lester and Robertson, 1995; Marshall, 1993; Rock, 1997; Rosbrow, 1997; J. Sarnat, 1992; Schindelheim, 1995; Strean, 1991; Teitelbaum, 1990; Wolkenfeld, 1990).

With the contemporary emphasis on the centrality of transference and countertransference in supervision, it is no longer possible to differentiate the supervisee's professional development from her personal growth, or her professional persona from her personality. Rather, the professional *is* the personal. In addition, to the extent that psychodynamic supervision is expected to model the theoretical approach being taught, relational supervision cannot be conducted effectively without addressing the supervisee's countertransference to her patient, her transference to the supervisor, and the supervisor's countertransferences to the patient and to the supervisee at more than a surface level. As James Fosshage (1997) puts it, "The analyst's experience of the patient is central in understanding and guiding the analytic process. Within this context, the 'teach/treat' dichotomy is no longer a meaningful distinction, for 'treating' corresponds with illuminating the analyst's experience, a necessary process for 'teaching' " (p. 202). If contemporary relational supervision is incompatible with a rigid demarcation between teaching and "treating," we need a model of supervision as a fully analytic process that, because it encompasses exploration of relational patterns alive in both the supervised treatment and in supervision, includes some blurring of teaching and "treating."

Perhaps first and foremost, a relational view of the teach/treat issue invites analysts to imagine the possibility that judicious, mutually negotiated interpenetration of what historically has been defined as teaching and "treating" in supervision vitally enhances the professional development of the supervisee. This requires analysts to reexamine all the reasons underlying the taboo against crossing the teach/treat line, including those embedded in the politics of power that often characterized the first century of psychoanalytic practice and supervision. In particular, it is helpful to revisit the notion that only the personal analyst can address the supervisee's psychodynamics. How much of this attitude really is in the interest of the supervisee versus a protection of the analyst's power as assumed and as assigned by the psychoanalytic guild? How much do analysts and supervisors deeply fear competing with one another, perhaps by offering a patient/supervisee different perspectives on a psychodynamic issue or relational theme? In this case, is a strict teach/treat barrier rationalized as protective of the patient/supervisee when, in fact, it primarily shields the analyst and supervisor from engaging with and processing their real and imagined relationship with one another? When defending the teach/treat boundary, how much do we unnecessarily infantilize the supervisee instead of mindfully joining with her to consider both her strengths and her vulnerabilities in supervision? Can we really teach contemporary approaches to psychoanalysis *without* at times engaging with supervisees in deeply personal explorations of their psychological processes? If not, how do we pay attention to their psychic functioning without inviting potentially intrusive or overzealous interpretations?

Donnel Stern (1997), in deconstructing the analytic endeavor, points out that most of us develop and live by "conventionalized narratives" that are the simplest and most natural accounts of our experiences. They become our unexamined truths. Similarly, during its first century of development, psychoanalysis developed certain conventional narratives about training that often are accepted unquestioningly, because doing so makes it easier to live our analytic lives. The teach/treat taboo is one of these conventionalized narratives. As Stern indicates, however, unreflective conformity to a conventionalized narrative involves a price:

> Conventional narratives, always the path of least resistance, are so seductively easy to slip into that we are seldom even aware of having chosen them. It is dismayingly easy, when one has some reason to reflect on one's experience in any particular moment, to find oneself hovering around the cultural mean, around predigested perceptions. (p. 140)

The demarcation of the teach/treat barrier in psychoanalytic supervision is one conventional activity that many analysts enact through embeddedness in their professional culture. Through often unconscious identification with their own supervisors, they themselves do not think through and devise a personal formulation of teaching and "treating" in supervision. It is, however, only through "imaginative, disembedding" (Stern, 1997, p. 25) reflection on the dilemma of teaching and "treating" in supervision that a contemporary conceptualization of this central supervisory dimension can be developed. When analyst, supervisor, and supervisee individually formulate as much as possible all the readily available and passively dissociated (Stern, 1997) reasons for and against blurring the teach/treat boundary, each then can arrive at a personal construction of teaching and "treating" that promises to maximize the supervisee's opportunity to learn the craft of psychoanalysis and, in doing so, to take well-considered yet, paradoxically, spontaneous risks.

If supervisors begin their supervisory encounters with articulated paradigms of that which is possible regarding teaching and "treating," they are more likely to negotiate with their supervisees a mutually influenced position that is imaginative and embedded in a shared understanding of what the supervisory dyad is about. Or supervisor and supervisee will learn early on that they are ill suited for each other in this crucial area and perhaps choose to part company without the shame, humiliation, and mystification too often accompanying supervisory "divorces."

ASSUMPTIONS OF THIS MODEL OF THE TEACH/TREAT ISSUE

In our discussion of the teach/treat issue, we use quotation marks when discussing the "treating" that occurs in supervision. We do this to stress that, although any one supervisory session that focuses on the supervisee's psychology might be difficult for an observer to distinguish from any one of the supervisee's analytic sessions, there is nonetheless a distinctive, ongoing difference in the tasks of the two relationships, one which the supervisor holds in mind throughout supervision. That difference is addressed next in our delineation of the first of several assumptions included in our paradigm of teaching and "treating" in supervision.

"Treating" Is Indentured to Teaching

One central tenet of a contemporary construction of the teach/treat issue is that supervision is most effective when supervisor and supervisee thoughtfully cooperate in ensuring that the "treat" aspect of supervision remains indentured to the overarching goal of facilitating the supervisee's growth as a clinician. Depending on the particular countertransference response of the supervisee to the patient, or of the supervisor to either the patient or the supervisee, and further depending on the nature of the supervisory relationship co-constructed by supervisor and supervisee, the depth and breadth of the "treating" aspect of supervision will vary greatly among supervisory dyads. Generally, however, exploration of the supervisee's countertransference to her patient and/or her transference to the supervisor is focused somewhat differently than in treatment. While in the analytic setting, the objective is to explore as fully as possible the genetic origins and range of potential meanings attributable to the transference–countertransference constellations emerging in the dyad, in supervision, discussion of the supervisee's psychological functioning and its impact on relational patterns at play in supervision and in the supervised treatment is more limited in scope. Here, the goal is for supervisee and supervisor to pursue the supervisee's personality and character only as far as is necessary to clarify the vicissitudes of the supervisory relationship and to promote effective psychoanalytic work with the supervised patient. An example illustrates typical application of this aspect of our model.

Laura was an experienced, quite gifted clinician working with

Susannah, a 19-year-old college student. In telling her supervisor, Jack, a little about herself early on in supervision, Laura mentioned having financed her undergraduate college education by working days and going to school at night. Her parents neither valued education nor were financially able to assist her with college expenses. It was clear to Jack that Laura, almost defiantly proud of her tenacious pursuit of education, was also angry and disappointed that her parents could neither afford to finance her education nor offer her much emotional support or encouragement.

Laura's work with Susannah went well for some months, during which Jack and Laura focused on the transference and countertransference paradigms at play in both the treatment and between them. Several months into supervision, however, Laura's tone of voice changed when she presented Susannah. At the time, therapist and patient had been examining the many extratherapeutic and transference meanings to Susannah's occasional shoplifting, abuse of alcohol, and overeating. Suddenly, instead of speaking about her patient in her characteristic measured but warm manner, Laura became impatient with and demeaning of her patient in supervision. Jack was puzzled until Laura revealed that Susannah had begun cutting classes at the prestigious college her parents paid for her to attend and was in danger of failing the semester. In one supervisory session, Laura derisively asked, "Can you believe this kid is cutting class just to have sex with her boyfriend because that's when he's available?" Instead of engaging with Susannah to analyze this behavior, Laura was conveying her dismay and disapproval of the class cutting.

At other times in the supervisory work, Laura had been open about exploring the meaning of her responses to both Susannah and Jack. Jack first commented that Laura seemed very angry with Susannah and wondered what might be happening in the transference and countertransference of the treatment to generate such an intense countertransference reaction. When Laura replied, she focused on her concern for Susannah and her worry that her patient would "blow such a great opportunity that's just been handed to her on a silver platter." Jack asked if there might be anything else about this form of acting out that particularly upset Laura. Laura became uncharacteristically defensive, pointing out that her patient's self-induced risk of failing a semester was good enough reason to be extremely frustrated with Susannah. As gently as possible, Jack then asked Laura if her strong reaction to her patient and to this particular form of acting out might stem, at least in part, from personal feelings about Susannah apparently blithely trashing what Laura would have cherished—a college education at a good school, paid for by parents who valued an education. Jack added that if he were Laura, he might want to shake some sense into Susannah. Instead of staying with her to better understand what this acting out was all about and what Susannah might be conveying about her relationship with her parents, her internalized constructions of self and other, and the transference toward Laura then active in the treatment, he might want just to tell her to grow up!

When Laura returned for the next supervisory session, she said she had been very angry at Jack for interpreting her reaction to Susannah as embedded in her own psychodynamics. In the meantime, however, she had brought the issue up in her psychoanalytic psychotherapy and found that her therapist thought Jack might be on to something worth exploring further. Somewhat ruefully, but with her sense of humor restored, Laura said that it was unlikely that both Jack and her therapist were totally off, so maybe she had some work to do. She asked Jack to help by letting her know if and when he heard this dynamic come into her clinical work again.

Here, we see a contained and circumscribed example of a blurred teach/treat boundary. Laura's envy toward Susannah, expressed through her derisive remarks and disapproving attitude, interfered with her work as a therapist. Jack's "treat" intervention focused on Laura's professional work. He and Laura did not go further into her relationship with her parents, nor did they talk about the possible ways in which this dynamic affected Laura's other relationships. However, Jack's interpretation was undeniably in the "treat" area, and it initially aroused defensiveness and resentment in Laura. Yet it apparently stimulated a deeper consideration of this aspect of Laura's psychological functioning in her own therapy, where it likely led to enhanced personal growth. In this vignette, "treating" in supervision remained indentured to the primary task of teaching while, in the supervisee's own treatment, the goal of personal development took priority.

Supervisees Can Limit the Extent of "Treating"

A second important component of our approach to the teach/treat issue is the supervisee's empowerment to limit the extent to which supervision focuses on her own psychology. Perhaps more than in any other realm of the supervisory process, the supervisee is empowered to define how deeply and broadly her psychic processes are available for mutual exploration in supervision. While supervisor and supervisee engage in mutual construction and ongoing negotiation of their relationship, the supervisee, in the end, must be able to draw the line on how therapeutic supervision becomes. An example makes the point.

Tom, a senior psychologist, focused closely on the relational patterns emerging both in clinical work and in the supervision of Lynn, a clinical psychology intern. Lynn remained in supervision with Tom for 2 years and, over the course of that time, shared much about her history and inner life. At one point, Lynn was working with a patient, Jean, who recently had reestablished a relationship with her mother, from whom she had been estranged for some time. The rapprochement was poignant, if imperfect, and followed long months of analytic work.

Jean's refinding her mother coincided with a period in Lynn's own analysis in which she was grieving deeply the difficult relationship she had with her own mother, whose death several years earlier precluded any possibility of repair and reunion. Without realizing it, Lynn was subtly undermining Jean's apparent success in reforming a relationship with her mother. When she and Tom listened to tapes of the therapy sessions with Jean, both could hear Lynn's lack of support for this development in her patient's life. In addition, the tapes made evident Jean's growing fear that in gaining back one mother, she would lose another. Tom wondered to Lynn about the possibility that she was having a very hard time letting Jean have her mother when she, Lynn, could not have her own. At that point, Lynn's analytic work with this issue was so intense that she felt too raw and tender to expose herself to her supervisor. She acknowledged to Tom that her pain about her mother was very alive then and that she was addressing it in treatment. Lynn told her supervisor that, at least for the time being, she needed to confine that work to her analysis. He immediately backed off, nodded his head in assent, and supported her by saying that he was sure she would get through what sounded like a rough time. Tom and Lynn then talked about interventions she could make in the clinical setting with Jean to let her know that Lynn would not abandon her if she continued a relationship with her mother.

In this vignette of Lynn's supervision with Tom, she felt empowered to limit the "treat" aspect of the supervisory relationship when it ventured into an area that she was not comfortable speaking about with her supervisor, even though it was a domain of her psychological functioning that interfered with her working optimally as an analyst. The supervisor, in turn, was respectful of Lynn's vulnerability and need for privacy. Their supervisory attention turned to more effective ways of working with Jean, without further discussion of the reasons that were leading Lynn to have trouble responding empathically to her patient. If, in a relational model of supervision, the teach/treat issue is to be flexibly negotiated and managed by each unique supervisory dyad, the supervisee needs to know that she is empowered to regulate the timing, pace, and depth of any exploration and interpretation of her own psychic processes. At the same time, the supervisor is free to introduce tactfully the possibility that a countertransference response has a personal aspect to it that might be useful to examine more closely.

In general, supervisees differ markedly in their desire to explore their own psyches analytically in supervision. Some supervisees are comfortable sharing a great deal of personal information and are open to examining rather fully with a supervisor the ways in which their own psychological functioning influences their clinical work. These supervisees may be enormously frustrated by a supervisor who maintains a strict teach/treat boundary. They may feel cheated out of what they consider to be the meat of a good supervisory experience. On the other hand, some therapists, especially, but not only, beginners, may be reluctant to delve much beyond the surface of their own psychology with a supervisor. These supervisees will feel frightened by and intruded on by a supervisor who, in the supervisee's subjective experience, too freely offers "treat" interventions during supervision. The expectations and preferred teach/treat style of each party, therefore, should be elaborated, and negotiated, to see if this is a supervisory dyad that can facilitate successful collaboration. The more advanced the supervisee, the more likely it is that she will have a clear idea of what she wants and expects in this area of supervision. Less experienced supervisees may need the supervisor to check in frequently with them to determine their level of comfort with whatever "treating" is occurring in the supervision.

While the supervisee is empowered to limit exploration of her psychodynamics and characteristic relational patterns, the supervisor is simultaneously responsible for keeping the supervisory process subordinated to the professional development of the supervisee, no matter how deeply supervisor and supervisee may explore the latter's psychology. A supervisee's focus on her psychic functioning, of course, can sometimes represent a defense against the anxiety of presenting clinical work. For example, to several supervisors over the course of a number of training years, one clinical psychology doctoral student seemed to defensively avoid presenting her clinical work, instead engaging her supervisors in endless conversations about the disorganizing effect on her of her parents' interminable divorce. In this case, the student was redirected to focus more on her work with patients and less on the more diffuse psychological distress she might be in at any given time, a matter much more appropriately taken up in her analysis.

Supervisor Self-Disclosure

A third assumption of this relational approach to teaching and "treating" in supervision involves the supervisor's willingness occasionally to make analytic observations about himself, as well as welcoming the supervisee's observations about the ways in which his personality affects the supervisory process. Much more than a therapist usually does, the supervisor can disclose ways in which his own psychodynamics, blind spots, and countertransference reactions have been problematic in his work as an analyst or as a supervisor. This use of the supervisor's self helps demystify and normalize the struggles every therapist faces when he contributes, wittingly and unwittingly, so much of his own personality to his clinical work. It also facilitates a more collegial atmosphere of mutuality and shared vulnerability than usually is achieved in treatment. An example illustrates this point.

Daniel, a clinical psychology doctoral student, began seeing several patients during his first year of training. In supervision, he repeatedly brought up feeling illegitimate in his new role. He had no right to be seeing patients; he did not know enough, he had little theoretical grounding, and he had just begun his own psychoanalysis. How could he help anyone? Daniel was concerned particularly that his patients were paying to see him, although he was able to acknowledge that the $5 clinic fee was very low.

Elena, Daniel's supervisor, suspected that her supervisee's sense of illegitimacy had a history of its own, but she felt that Daniel was too new at being a patient, a therapist, and a supervisee for her to make a "treat" comment or inquiry at that point in his training. Instead, Elena told Daniel about starting her private practice shortly after she was licensed as a psychologist. Despite her credentials, she told Daniel that she still had doubted her legitimacy to practice and was highly conflicted about being paid for her services. Elena mentioned to Daniel that her feelings about entering practice were partly typical, new therapist experiences and partly stemmed from elements of her personal history and psychodynamics, including insecurities about her general value that had not been completely worked through at the start of her career. She then shared with Daniel that, when her first private patient asked about her fee during their initial phone contact, Elena had mumbled the number, immediately adding that they could negotiate a lower fee if the patient could not afford to pay more. Daniel looked stunned and then began to laugh. Although he continued to struggle with feeling like a fraud with his patients, he had greater perspective on his experience and could have a sense of humor about it.

Here, Elena made a self-disclosing remark about her own inner life and its impact on her work. Essentially, she used herself as a metaphor to address indirectly Daniel's anxieties about his value and legitimacy. In exposing some of her own vulnerability as a new clinician, Elena helped Daniel to be more comfortable with his own, and she modeled an acceptance of the limitations we all face as analysts, as supervisors, and as supervisees.

While some focus on the supervisee's personal issues and psychology are inevitable in contemporary psychodynamic supervision, negotiation of the teach/treat issue in supervision may take a different course depending on whether or not the supervisee is in concurrent treatment.

WHEN THE SUPERVISEE IS IN CONCURRENT TREATMENT

Although a relational model of supervision usually results in some exploration of the supervisee's dynamics and relational themes, the approach suggested here creates space for an admixture of what has been called teaching and "treating" rather than dictating its inevitable occurrence in every supervision. Sometimes, the traditionally advocated division of labor between supervision and analysis suffices for a supervisee working through a conflict affecting both her personal and professional functioning. An example makes this point.

Alice, a fourth-year postdoctoral fellow, found both her work and her psychological equilibrium disrupted when she moved from subleased space to her own office. Although the new office was spacious and well located, it was less elegant, more poorly soundproofed, and less private than the previous space. Because this was the first time Alice had had her own office, she felt keenly that it represented her. Its limitations were thus a source of acute anxiety for her.

One of Alice's patients, Henry, had experienced the analyst's office as Alice's body throughout their work and so reacted to the move with intense distress. Unconsciously, Henry felt that he had been pushed out of Alice's body because of his intrusive and demanding presence. Furthermore, Henry interpreted the differences between the old and new office as persecutory impingements. In his first session in the new office, Henry vehemently attacked everything about it. Alice, already anxious and doubtful about her new space, responded countertransferentially to Henry with guilt and intensified anxiety.

The day after this difficult session with Henry, Alice discussed the office change in both supervision and analysis. Alice's supervisor, Warren, talked about the various meanings offices come to assume for both analysts and patients. He normalized Alice's anxiety about the new office space. Warren also shared his own sense of disruption when he had changed offices over the years and reassured Alice that the sense of impingement would decrease for her and her patients as the weeks passed. Then, Warren and Alice focused more specifically on Henry's response to the move and Alice's countertransference reactions to Henry, elaborating the material to clarify further the transference and countertransference paradigm currently in play between analyst and patient. Alice felt joined with and supported by Warren, more able to think about what the move had meant to her patient and, thus, more confident about working with the relational material currently alive in Henry's treatment.

In analysis, Alice explored her personal responses to the move, including her worries about the inadequacies of the new space, and her reactions to Henry's attacking comments. Here, Alice elaborated, with intense anxiety, her experience of her devalued office-body, a representation of her female self, unworthy of respect or professional esteem. Simultaneously, she became aware of her concomitant idealization of her male analyst's calm, solid, seemingly more admirable office-body. Alice experienced her analyst as the grounded, containing mother as well as the competent, bodily intact father she neither had within her nor felt she could become. Alice's painful experience of the contrast between her experience of herself and her idealization of her analyst were worked through over the course of several difficult sessions, resulting in a marked decrease in her anxiety about her new office.

In this example, the supervisor–supervisee and supervisee/patient–analyst dyads divided work on the personal and professional impact of Alice's new office in a traditional way. In supervision, Alice and Warren addressed the material primarily with Alice's professional learning in mind, and Warren provided needed support. In analysis, Alice examined more deeply and elaborated more fully the anxieties and unconscious fantasies evoked by both her move and Henry's devaluing remarks. In keeping with other models of teaching and "treating," the supervisor addressed the effect of Alice's anxiety on her work with patients, especially Henry, while her analyst focused with her on the source of her anxiety as well as its broader meanings in terms of her experiences of self and other.

One reason the traditional teach/treat model worked so well for Alice, her supervisor, and analyst was Alice's acute awareness that her office situation upset her on many levels. Conscious that her countertransference response to Henry was at least partly embedded in her own psychodynamics, Alice was able to introduce the material in both supervision and psychoanalysis in different but ultimately related ways. Because this supervisee already was aware of the dynamic underpinnings of a countertransference response, she was able to pursue it independently in both the supervisory and treatment dyads.

Sometimes, however, a realm of the supervisee/patient's psychodynamic functioning assumes prominence in supervision at a time when the supervisee's treatment is too centrally involved with something else to shift gears. Here, it could be disruptive to the patient's personal growth, the primary goal of treatment, to expect the therapeutic process to explore a dynamic, conflict, self or other representation, or relational striving that is impeding the supervisee's professional growth. In this situation, the integrity of the supervisee's treatment precludes examination of the personal issue interfering with her work as a clinician, at least at the time that the issue is salient for that work. At junctures like these, analyst, patient/supervisee, and supervisor can decide within their respective dyads whether or not the supervisory pair might focus productively on the supervisee's psychology to the extent that such analytic work within supervision promotes the supervisee's professional competence and confidence. An example illustrates this possibility.

Ilene, a senior analyst, supervised Marion, a third-year postdoctoral psychoanalytic candidate, who was also in her fourth year of analysis with Paula, another senior analyst. Marion had been severely attacked and abandoned by her alcoholic father, who was widowed shortly after Marion's birth. Throughout Marion's childhood, her father flew into drunken rages, during which he viciously blamed her for all that was wrong in his own life. Often, these attacks were followed by extended business trips, during which Marion's father neither telephoned nor wrote to his daughter, leaving her in the care of a nanny. Marion began her analysis with a pronounced sense of herself as fundamentally wrong, unlovable, unwantable, and toxic. She also feared that any kind of self-assertion could evoke murderous rage and abandonment by another, so she tended to be unendingly tolerant of others, even when their behavior was in some way hostile.

Vivian, the patient Marion presented to Ilene, also had been traumatized as a child. Vivian's father, a successful and quite narcissistic politician, viewed his daughter primarily as an extension of his own organization of self. If she defied or disappointed him in any way, Vivian's father vilified her as ugly, stupid, and low class, then gave her the cold shoulder for days on end.

As Ilene and Marion discussed the latter's work with Vivian, Ilene realized that the therapeutic dyad was enacting a relational paradigm that was salient for both patient and therapist. Vivian, unconsciously identifying with her brutal father but subjectively experiencing herself as a wounded victim, regularly but subtly heaped contempt on Marion. For example, guessing from her drawl that Marion was a Southerner, Vivian regaled her with tales of the Civil War heroes populating her Yankee family, indicating to her therapist how much those ancestors had enjoyed crushing their Southern counterparts. Within the transference–countertransference of the treatment, Marion unconsciously identified with herself as a child and helplessly absorbed her patient's blows, while subjectively experiencing herself as incompetent and toxic to her patient.

Clearly, the relational paradigm at play in the treatment was reflective of psychodynamics and internalized relational configurations central for the patient, Vivian. Unfortunately, however, elements of

Marion's internalized relational world also were vitalized in her work with Vivian, through complex and rapidly shifting projective and introjective processes involving identifications with and self-organizations of victim, abuser, neglectful and neglected one, rescuer and rescued one. The sadomasochistic dance enacted by therapist and patient could be worked through successfully only when Marion experienced her patient's brutality and stood up to it instead of collapsing. For Marion, however, that evoked the possibility of becoming the abuser herself, an organization of self, representing an identification with her father, that she feared and despised.

In supervision, Ilene and Marion worked for some time on elaborating and understanding the patient's internal world and its elements being enacted in the treatment. At this point, their discussions of Marion's countertransference pertained to its context in Vivian's history, and conscious and dissociated relational patterns. Supervisor and supervisee addressed the need to make explicit, at some point, Vivian's identification with her father in her ruthlessness toward her therapist. During these supervisory sessions with Ilene, Marion seemed to go blank. Although she shook her head in agreement with Ilene, she appeared unable to marshal her own usually keen clinical insight and was affectively flat.

As the clinical work with Vivian and the supervision progressed, Ilene realized that Marion's countertransference responses to Vivian's verbal sadism and her inability to make use of her supervisor's interventions were as much related to the supervisee's own history and psychodynamics as they were to the specifics of Vivian's unfolding typical relational patterns in the treatment. Ilene was concerned that Marion's paralysis and emotional deadness in the face of a patient's sadistic attacks could limit her effectiveness as an analyst with not only Vivian but also with other patients who might unconsciously detect this vulnerability in their therapist. At the same time, Ilene worried about being experienced by Marion as blaming and intrusive if she made any links between her supervisee's clinical work and her history; perhaps she would seem to validate Marion's perception of herself as toxic and incompetent. In the end, Ilene decided that it was more respectful of Marion to share some of her thoughts than to remain silent.

In the next supervisory session, Ilene asked Marion if she had considered the possibility that, in addition to enacting with Vivian a core relational dynamic in the patient's psychological repertoire, she also was, perhaps unconsciously, reexperiencing something about her own relationship with her verbally annihilating and abandoning father. Marion had not thought about this before and grew visibly anxious when Ilene introduced the idea. She asked the supervisor what she thought might be going on, and Ilene answered that it seemed at least possible to her that Marion might unconsciously be reacting to Vivian as she once did to her father's rages; that is, as a terrified, helpless child who felt paralyzed by but responsible for her father–patient's attacks. Marion replied that she could feel herself shutting down right then and there with Ilene and knew that this was one characteristic strategy she employed to close out pain and, especially, anger. Ilene said she would like to work with this material in whatever way might be most helpful to Marion and to her work with patients. Marion told Ilene she would think about it and let her know.

Marion and Paula, her analyst, then spoke about Marion's supervision and about the countertransference responses she was experiencing toward Vivian. They also sorted through the many reactions Marion had to Ilene's comments. The analytic pair agreed that although the material evoked in the clinical work with Vivian and in Marion's supervision was crucial, calling for their analytic attention at some point, the analysis at that point was attending to equally important but quite different matters. Moreover, Marion's analytic treatment was embedded in transference and countertransference configurations that would not accommodate easily to exploration and working through of Marion's relational response to a brutal attack from another. Specifically, the most salient transference–countertransference matrix at play in Marion's analysis was her experience of Paula as the available, alive mother she never had. Marion and her analyst agreed that since the dynamic of a vicious attack from another was primed in Marion's supervision, perhaps she could pursue it further there, to the extent that she and her supervisor felt comfortable.

During the next supervisory session, Marion told Ilene that she agreed that her countertransference experience of Vivian's assaults was indeed partly embedded in her own psychodynamics. Marion acknowledged that her vulnerability to such barrages affected her clinical work as an analyst with Vivian and with other patients. She explained that she and her analyst had discussed the matter and were not prepared to engage this issue right now, and asked Ilene if they could continue to address it in supervision. Ilene agreed and over the next few months together they collaborated to help Marion articulate the dissociated feelings, body states, thoughts, and fantasies she experienced when faced with another person's equally dissociated but potent rage. The supervisor was supportive of Marion, telling her how difficult it would be for anyone with her history to process in the moment and adequately respond to the kind of vicious verbal assaults Vivian regularly launched. She encouraged Marion to imagine unfreezing with both her father and Vivian and, further, to envision a nonparalytic response to either or both of them. Eventually, Marion was able to experience how truly furious she was at her father–patient for projecting their own terrified and terrifying states into her. She realized that, as a child, she had little choice but to absorb and identify with her father's projections, but as an adult, she was getting sick of acquiescing to Vivian's projective activities.

As the supervisory year went on, Marion was less disabled by Vivian's attacks and could even begin playfully narrating the "Civil War" going on in the consultation room, where, with ever so civil an outward appearance, Vivian waged bitter war against her analyst's effectiveness. Still later, patient and analyst bantered about whether a given session was a "Chancellorsville," where the Yankees were slaughtered, a "Gettysburg," where the Johnny Rebs were routed, or an "Appomattox," where mutual respect and repair seemed imaginable for a time to both North and South.

This supervision clearly evolved into an analytic process in which Marion's personal issues were addressed quite deeply. Links were made between Marion's countertransference to Vivian and her relationship with her own father. The supervisee was encouraged to elaborate her feelings and fantasies when hit with a verbal barrage. She was asked to imagine alternative states of self, affects, and responses to an assaultive other. Verbatim transcripts of some supervisory sessions would be hard to differentiate from transcripts of some therapy sessions. At the same time, the focus of the analytic process taking place in supervision remained fixed on Marion's growing freedom and effectiveness as an analytic practitioner, specifically, in her clinical work not only with the supervised patient but also with other patients. In her analysis, Marion eventually revisited this dynamic even more broadly and deeply, with a full complement of transference and countertransference manifestations alive between herself and her analyst. Yet it is inescapably true that the analytic exploration of Marion's relational themes in supervision resulted in significant personal growth for the supervisee that was indistinguishable from her professional development. Here, Ilene, Marion, and Paula negotiated a way of working "together," albeit in their respective dyads, which allowed Marion's supervision to initiate a working through of an important relational pattern that affected many domains of Marion's life. In the system comprised of patient–analyst/supervisee (Vivian–Marion), supervisee–supervisor (Marion–Ilene), and supervisee/patient–analyst (Marion–Paula), the mutually negotiated, respectfully enacted blurring of teaching and "treating" successfully generated a creative, liberating approach to very old problems for both Vivian and Marion.

It is this kind of interdyadic collaboration about analytic engagement of the supervisee's psychology in supervision that other models of supervision have warned against. The paradigm presented in this vignette admittedly challenges both analyst and supervisor to negotiate the holding capacity and work space of each analytic setting to preserve its unique integrity. It also asks them to attend to and internally process feelings toward one another, including competitive ones, that can arise when the supervisory dyad blurs teaching and "treating." On the other hand, analysts and supervisors often experience myriad reactions toward one another even if there is no overt discussion of the supervisee's psychology in supervision. They, too, develop transferences to one another based on actual acquaintance, reputation, or reports from their shared patient/supervisee. Our model of the teach/treat issue, in fact, may mitigate against more pernicious, covert enactments of the supervisor's and analyst's feelings about each other by opening up in each dyad potentially clarifying discussions of the supervisee's expectations and experience of each analytic relationship. Here, the supervisor and analyst are more likely to attempt to consciously process and better understand reactions toward one another that might otherwise be acted out in ways that are mystifying or destructive for the patient/supervisee.

Another kind of blurring of the therapeutic and supervisory roles can occur when the supervisee develops and enacts with the supervisor a transference and countertransference paradigm not at that time alive in his analysis. Other models of supervision commonly warn that a supervisee's personal analysis can be impeded if he displaces onto the supervisor transference phenomena better projected onto, enacted with, and interpreted by the trainee's personal analyst. In addition, there has been concern that if a supervisor engages with a supervisee to analyze transference manifestations arising in the supervision, a destructive competition between the supervisor and the supervisee's analyst could ensue. For the most part, supervisors have been advised to refrain from commenting on, much less engaging with such transference phenomena, and/or they have been admonished to refer the candidate back to his personal analysis to work on that transference.

Recently, dissenting voices (Fosshage, 1997; Harris & Ragen, 1995; Issacharoff, 1984; Lester and Robertson, 1995; Marshall, 1993) have pointed out that a supervisee's personal analysis follows it own course, which cannot be expected to change just because an important aspect of his internalized relational world has been activated in another relationship. Furthermore, instructing a supervisee to take a transference to the supervisor, or a countertransference response to a patient back to her analysis, ignores the co-creation of the supervisee's reactions within the patient–therapist and supervisee–supervisor dyads. How can we teach that a patient's verbalizations, fantasies, affects, and relational strivings toward the analyst are co-constructed by the supervisee and her patient if we do not then commit ourselves as supervisors to exploring with the supervisee his verbalizations, fantasies, affects, and relational strivings toward the patient and the supervisor as co-constructed within the treatment and supervisory dyads? And if we accept that all these dyads exert mutual influence on one another, and thus on supervisory material, it is inconsistent to exclude from mutually negotiated discussions of that material anything deemed "too therapeutic." To do so creates a contradiction between the message and the medium that is at least mystifying and can be experienced as humiliating to the supervisee. Indeed, it often is far more disruptive to the supervisee's personal analysis, as well as to his supervision, to expect the analytic dyad to address a personal conflict or relational configuration emerging in supervision than it is for the supervisor and supervisee to take up the issue within the relationship in which it arises, even if that blurs the teach/treat line.

The following example, taken from the postdoctoral training of one of us (Frawley-O'Dea, 1998), illustrates a subtle blurring of teaching and "treating" that occurred around a specific transference–countertransference constellation alive within the supervision and not at play within her analysis. This may at first read like a quite frequently occurring idealization of a supervisor. It is, however, the supervisor's overt acknowledgment of the supervisee's transference and his willingness to play with her within a particular transference and countertransference constellation that imbues this supervisory relationship with a slight blurring of the teach/treat line guarded against in other models of supervision.

During one postdoctoral supervision, I (Frawley-O'Dea) developed a transference to my supervisor as a romantic, oedipal father. At the time, my primary transference to my male analyst was as a soothing, consistently nurturing mother. In supervision, there were a number of exchanges that conveyed my transference to my supervisor, and he acknowledged his awareness of and willingness to engage with those relational strivings. During one supervisory session, for example, I gave my supervisor a number of "gifts," specifically reminiscences about the helpfulness of several of his past clinical suggestions. That my comments were more personally and psychologically meaningful than the idealization often felt by supervisees toward their supervisors was indicated by their delivery in a sweet, girlish voice to a father I adored, and whose words I hung on. Shortly after this series of shyly offered compliments, I told my supervisor that I was finding my clinical work to be much more fun since beginning *therapy* with him. I stopped, blushing, and said, "I mean supervision," to which he playfully responded, "Well, whatever we are doing here," and we both giggled as if sharing a delicious yet slightly dangerous secret. At the end of the supervisory period, I gave my supervisor a kaleidoscope that consciously represented for me the variety of perspectives he could bring to clinical material. As he lifted the kaleidoscope from its box, he held it up and exclaimed, "Oh, like a spyglass." I responded, "Gee, my father was a sea captain." The supervisor smiled, shrugged, and said, "Well, there you go."

During the time I worked with this supervisor, I spoke with my analyst about my oedipal experience in supervision, and my analyst delighted in it with me. At that juncture in my analysis, my analyst conveyed little more than his support for my relationship with my supervisor, commenting once, for instance, how wonderfully special it must be to feel that I was learning so much at the same time that I was enjoying a romance. In this situation, it was clear to me, my analyst, and my supervisor, that my supervisor and I were enacting an oedipal transference and countertransference constellation that coexisted with our grown-up supervisory collaboration. It was important to me to know that the supervisor knew what was happening between us at the level of play and illusion, and that he accepted and even enjoyed it. He, in turn, conveyed his awareness and willingness to participate in my oedipal fantasy, although we never discussed explicitly the genetic history, internalized relational organization, or even the profound meaning the experience had for me. Those elaborations and that meaning making were reserved for a much later period in my analysis, when they became salient within that relationship. At the time of supervision, my analyst "simply" supported and took pleasure in this extra-analytic transference and countertransference matrix, enacting a delighted and securely indulgent mother of an oedipal daughter.

In retrospect, I think it would have been both terribly hurtful and an impediment to personal and professional development alike had my supervisor rejected or overtly interpreted my oedipal yearnings, or had my analyst interpreted their expression within the supervision as resistance or as harmful in some other way to my analysis. Instead, my supervisor and analyst allowed me to work with them simultaneously on several important professional and psychological projects, spanning multiple developmental stages, bespeaking quite different degrees of regression, and giving external life to a number of disparate, internalized self and object paradigms. Throughout the supervision, however, my professional growth remained paramount, and the oedipal enactments served it well. Coexisting with whatever personal development the oedipal relationship with my supervisor fostered, I also found myself appreciating more keenly the tenderness of my own patient's oedipal feelings.

The vignettes presented here suggest that the interpenetration of teaching and "treating" can result in enhanced personal and professional growth for the supervisee. Each set of supervisory and analytic dyads will arrive at their own uniquely constructed and, one hopes, flexible position regarding what is spoken about in each dyad and to what extent the supervisory relationship will be available to and welcomed by the trainee to name and explore personal issues. No matter where each pair of dyads ends up, a relational model of teaching and "treating" in supervision ensures that the very delimiting of that dimension itself becomes a mutually constructed, analytic experience. A slightly different scenario arises when the supervisee is not concurrently in treatment: How, then, is the teach/treat issue negotiated?

WHEN THE SUPERVISEE IS NOT
IN CONCURRENT TREATMENT

Finding an appropriate and comfortable teach/treat boundary often is an even more challenging and delicate task when the supervisee is not currently, or never has been, in treatment. When the supervisee is in her own therapy or analysis, there is a container for her psychological exploration and a process in which her personal development goes forward. As teaching and "treating" blur in supervision, both supervisor and supervisee can rely on the supervisee's analytic relationship to provide support for any analytic work initiated in supervision. Moreover, in the best of all worlds, the analytic dyad participates in defining whatever "treating" occurs in supervision. When the supervisee is not in concurrent treatment, however, it is left to the supervisor and supervisee to negotiate the degree to which the supervisee's psychology can become a focus of supervisory attention without undermining as the primary goal of supervision the supervisee's professional development. The outcome of these negotiations may be quite different when the supervisee has never been in treatment or she has completed a personal analysis.

When the Supervisee Has Never Been in Treatment

Most clinicians would agree that involvement in personal therapy is a de facto credential for a psychotherapist and, of course, analytic training requires a personal analysis. It can happen, however, that supervisors working with clinicians early on in their training, or consulting privately with practitioners in their communities, encounter individuals who are not and have never been in their own therapies or analyses. Exploration of countertransferences to patients, a supervisory endeavor that almost always occurs at the teach/treat intersection, may evoke a myriad of complicated affects, self-states, fantasies, and relational strivings in the supervisee. Depending on the personality and psychological organization of the particular supervisee, the intensity of these phenomena may interfere with the learning task. Furthermore, the supervisee who has no experience with therapy may develop transferences to the supervisor with little insight into their origin or meaning. It is probable, therefore, that in most supervisions with clinicians who have not yet been in treatment, work on the supervisee's countertransference will be more circumscribed than with supervisees who are or have been patients. In these supervisions, identification and limited exploration of the personal issues underlying the supervisee's countertransference responses to the supervised patient and transference reactions to the supervisor can crystallize for the supervisee the importance of a personal therapeutic experience. The following vignette illustrates the complexity and the possibility in supervisory work with a supervisee who has never been in treatment.

Bea, a mature, third-year clinical psychology doctoral student, had accumulated extensive prior human services experience. In their first session, she told Deirdre, her supervisor, that she had never been in treatment but very much wanted to begin therapy when her finances would allow it. In their first supervisory session, Bea also commented that after the completion of her previous successful practicum experience, she no longer felt that she was dealing with issues of "basic trust," in Erikson's (1963) terms, and hoped that this supervision would allow her to engage her issues around "initiative versus shame and guilt." Deirdre was not sure what to make of that statement, but she filed it away for consideration at a later time. As their work began, she found Bea to be bright, motivated, highly skilled for her level of training, and quite likable.

Early on in supervision, Bea came to a session and reported having felt criticized by Deirdre in the previous session. She said this with great anxiety and was clearly angry and in pain over what she perceived to be her supervisor's harshness toward her. Deirdre, not conscious of having felt critical toward Bea, was surprised by her reaction but let Bea know that she would reflect on what quite evidently had been a disruptive session for her supervisee.

In the following session, Bea said that *she* had reflected on her reactions to Deirdre and concluded that her experience of her supervisor as critical had been a projection of feelings she was having in other relationships in her life. Now, Bea was grateful that Deirdre had *not* been critical of her in the previous session when she expressed angry feelings! At this point, Deirdre wondered whether her supervisee unconsciously was trying to undo what she feared might have been a damaging attack on the supervisory relationship, or whether, in fact, she had come to see Deirdre differently. Since Bea was not and never had been in therapy, Deirdre could not be sure that Bea had a space other than the supervisory relationship where such distressing feelings could be further explored and contained. For this reason, Deirdre was also reluctant to verbalize her musings about their relationship so far.

Over the next several months, Deirdre became concerned that Bea backed off and shared nothing more about her perceptions of the supervisory relationship. Meanwhile, Bea did become curious about her countertransference experiences and offered her thoughts about aspects of her own psychology that might be influencing her work with patients. These reflections suggested Bea's deep commitment to her growth as a clinician. Finally, Deirdre asked Bea how she felt things were going between them in supervision. Bea seemed flustered and deflected the question by stating simply that she was learning alot. Again unsure about how far to push her, or what Bea's reluctance to disclose more about her feelings about the supervisory relationship meant, Deirdre let it go.

In the same supervisory session, Bea presented her work with Grace, an extremely socially inhibited young woman, who described her father as vaguely sexually inappropriate. Six months into her weekly therapy, Grace began describing sexual fantasies in some detail. Bea had felt uneasy during that therapy session and, as she and Deirdre discussed it in supervision, Bea realized that she found Grace's presentation of her fantasies seductive. In turn, Bea was concerned that her own inquiries about Grace's fantasies also were vaguely seductive, and worried that she might be colluding with her patient in a sexualized enactment. Perhaps because of her discomfort in the treatment hour, Bea had offered Grace an intellectualized interpretation at a moment when a more affectively oriented response might have been more useful. When Deirdre noted this, Bea expressed frustration with herself, saying, "It seems like I *often* step back just when my patients most need me to be there emotionally. I just let them down in that way and I don't understand it. It's this kind of issue that makes me wish I were in therapy." Deirdre suggested that they try to understand more about why Bea might have backed off from Grace at this particular moment.

After discussing the material of the session further, Deirdre and Bea formulated that Grace longed to be closer to Bea but feared that her erotically tinged yearnings were dangerous and would result in boundary transgressions if she expressed them directly to Bea. Bea had resonated unconsciously with Grace's concern in the countertransference; she therefore responded by stepping back with a "safely" intel-lectualized interpretation.

But clarification of this specific transference and countertransfer-ence enactment did not fully address Bea's concerns. "I back off from emotionally loaded material with other patients, too. Why is that? How does a therapist become comfortable with intensely affective material?" Deirdre reminded Bea that she, Bea, had not yet worked on such mate-rial with a therapist of her own. Deirdre told Bea that such work un-doubtedly would increase her comfort with her patients' affects. Deirdre also shared with Bea that her own analysis had been a tremendously im-portant part of both her personal and professional growth. She added that most people who enter this "impossible profession" do so, at least in part, because their own parents failed in some way to respond adequately to their emotional states and relational longings.

As Deirdre spoke, Bea's eyes welled with tears, but she said noth-ing. Deidre did not address Bea's tears at that moment, sensing that to do so might make Bea feel self-conscious. A few minutes later, how-ever, when Bea had regained her composure, Deirdre asked her if she would like to share something about her tears. When Bea spoke, a tor-rent of pent up thoughts and feelings spilled out. Weeping, Bea de-scribed struggling with strong feelings she had been having toward Deirdre and had tried to suppress. For instance, she sometimes found herself thinking about Deirdre between sessions and wishing that they could spend more time together. Because she was not in therapy, Bea feared that she would try to use Deirdre as a therapist and thus trans-gress their relationship's appropriate limits. Furthermore, her early, sudden, intensely negative experience of Deirdre, which she believed to be a distortion, frightened her. She worried that powerful uncon-scious reactions to her supervisor could get out of control and jeopar-dize her relationship with Deirdre. Like her patient, Bea feared that expressing intense feelings to someone important to her could result only in broken boundaries and a ruined relationship.

Bea went on to say that she had filled up with tears when Deirdre mentioned parents. She reported that her mother's communication of a sense of her own feelings of inferiority had distressed her deeply. Bea realized that she had felt a great pressure to be perfect for her mother, and also for Deirdre, to protect them both from such distressing feel-ings, and that she felt great feelings of shame and humiliation when she did not succeed in doing so. Bea's initial request to Deirdre for help with the issue of initiative versus shame and guilt now became

understandable, as well as her early sensitivity to "criticism" of her im-
perfections, and her subsequent anxious reaction when she began to
talk about all of that to Deirdre. She feared that Deirdre, like her
mother, could not handle such upsetting feelings, because Deirdre
might be as vulnerable as her mother had been to feelings of inadequacy.

Deirdre told Bea that it was moving to her that Bea took the risk
of displaying so much vulnerability within their relationship. Deirdre
tried to normalize some of Bea's experience by stating that supervision
often evokes powerful feelings in both supervisor and supervisee. In
addition, Deirdre validated how unsettling all that can be for the
supervisee, especially if she is not in a treatment relationship in which
she can explore the origins and multiple meanings of her reactions.
Finally, Deirdre proposed that, as their supervisory work progressed,
she and Bea could continue to discuss their own experiences of the supervisory relationship, especially as they related to the supervised case
material.

During the rest of the supervision, Deirdre and Bea continued to
examine Bea's countertransference responses, identifying a number of
recurrent themes. While the supervisory dyad occasionally ventured
into the personal meaning of these relational predispositions for Bea,
Deirdre usually refrained from joining her supervisee in any more than
a surface exploration of the material and, rather, restated how much
Bea's own therapy would enrich her ability to understand, fully feel,
and work with her own psychodynamics. At the end of their time together, as they processed their feelings about the supervisory experience, Bea stated that she had begun to gather information about low-
cost analysis.

The supervisory work with Bea illustrates the delicacy of supervising someone who has never been in treatment. The clinical and supervisory processes evoke regressions and stir up myriad powerful, sometimes mystifying and frightening thoughts, affects, fantasies, body
states, self and other representations, or organizations of self in the
supervisee. Yet the supervisee who is not in concurrent treatment has
no one with whom to engage, whose primary goal is to enhance her
personal psychological development. The supervisee's countertransferences to patients and transferences to the supervisor, therefore, may
strain the capacity of the supervisory dyad to hold them without relinquishing the learning task. Bea intuitively appreciated the potential
difficulties involved in bringing the full intensity of her transference

reactions to the supervisor into the work of the supervisory dyad, especially since she was not in concurrent treatment. Yet withholding them was also disruptive. With more naive supervisees, or with those having more serious psychological difficulties, the supervisory dyad may not be able to engage in both teaching and attending analytically to the supervisee's psychodynamics in a way that is useful to the supervisee's professional development. Rather, the supervisor may have to limit herself to didactic teaching, while more aggressively recommending personal treatment for the supervisee.

An important addendum to this account of the work between Bea and Deirdre raises yet another element of complexity to working with the supervisee who is not in treatment. When Bea later reflected on her terminated supervisory relationship with Deirdre, she became aware for the first time that feelings of shame and inadequacy about not being in psychotherapy had complicated their relationship. Bea realized that her tendency to feel that she was defective or inadequate—just as her mother had felt—had inhibited her participation in the supervision. She had been unable to know about or to speak about this anxiety with Deirdre during the supervision, because it was too loaded to bring into their relationship, and Deirdre had not understood this issue either. Bea had thus been caught in a double bind: Because she was not in psychotherapy at the time, her lack of a therapist not only became a source of feelings of inadequacy, but she also had no therapist to help her to process those feelings, so that she could then bring them safely back to Deirdre! This retrospective supervisee reflection serves as a reminder of the supervisor's inevitable limitations in fully understanding the impact of her supervisory participation upon her supervisees. Supervisors need their supervisees to tell them how they have experienced their supervisor's interventions and, of course, it is the supervisor's responsibility to do all that is possible to create an environment within supervision where such disclosure is possible. Nonetheless, supervisees who lack the support of a treatment relationship may be less able to provide this feedback than those who are currently in treatment, or who have been in treatment.

When the Supervisee Has Completed Treatment

The supervisee who has terminated her personal treatment is different from the one who is in concurrent therapy or analysis, or who has never been in treatment. Like the latter, the supervisee currently does not have a therapeutic relationship to which to bring psychodynamic conflicts or relational responses emerging in either the supervised treatment or the supervision. In many cases, however, this supervisee has developed a self-analytic process through which she is able to contain and further analyze personal issues arising within the supervised treatment and the supervisory relationship. Here, the supervisee's analytic relationship is internalized and remains available to her as a now self-encapsulated vehicle for continued self-exploration and personal growth. As supervision progresses, the supervisor and supervisee develop a sense of how much "treating" the supervisory dyad can pursue without overburdening the supervisee's self-analytic capabilities or undermining the primary learning task of the supervision.

When the supervisee does not have well-developed self-analytic skills, or when personal issues emerge that evoke such regressive or previously unanalyzed material that seemingly requires further psychotherapeutic work, little blurring of teaching and "treating" may be possible within the context of the supervisory dyad, at least until the supervisee has returned to treatment. Here, the supervisory dyad is in a position similar to that in which the supervisee never has been analyzed. Supervisory exploration of the supervisee's countertransference to patients or transference to the supervisor may remain at the surface of the supervisee's psyche, particularly if the supervisory dyad determines that the supervisee is becoming overwhelmed or increasingly defensive.

The supervisor in this situation has an even more delicate challenge than the supervisor of a trainee not yet in treatment. A supervisee who has ended a therapy or analysis, especially with the agreement of her analyst, may be quite disrupted by the suggestion that, in fact, her analytic work was not "completed." Such a notion threatens the supervisee's perhaps hard-won identity as psychologically "healthy." Just as painful, the supervisee's trust in her former analyst may be shaken, causing her to question all the work and all the gains she relied on their having made together. Being perceived by the supervisor as someone needing further treatment, either with her former analyst or with someone new, often is a profoundly painful and disorienting injury to the supervisee's sense of herself. On the other hand, if the supervisee herself has concerns about lingering unanalyzed or insufficiently worked-through psychodynamic material, the supervisor's suggestion that further treatment might be helpful may be validating, albeit terribly painful and disappointing as well.

In this situation, it is helpful for the supervisor to note that many clinicians engage in any number of treatments in their lives and careers and that, often, it is not apparent that more analysis is needed until the patient reaches a new developmental crossroads that evokes previously dormant psychic material. If the supervisor has pursued more than one psychoanalysis or course of therapy, he can share that with the supervisee, perhaps commenting on how his different therapeutic experiences furthered his growth in different ways.

Once a supervisor suggests to a supervisee that a return to treatment is advisable, the transference–countertransference matrix of the supervisory dyad is bound to be affected in some way that may even parallel the supervisee's clinical work. For instance, a supervisee nursing a narcissistic wound may defensively withdraw in supervision, while becoming critical of patients in her work with them, projecting her vulnerable but unacceptable self onto them and identifying with her supervisor's perceived persecutory self. It is important for the supervisor and for the supervisory dyad to identify and, as much as possible, work through the relational fallout from the supervisor's suggestion that the trainee return to treatment. On occasion, this working through cannot be accomplished and the members of the supervisory dyad may decide to terminate their relationship, as illustrated in the following vignette.

Bernie was a third-year postdoctoral fellow who ended his psychoanalysis shortly before beginning supervision with Carolyn, a senior supervisor in his training program. After several months of supervisory work, Bernie said that he needed to process intensely negative feelings he experienced toward Carolyn, feelings that coexisted with respect and admiration for her clinical skills. Carolyn, open to that kind of supervisory material, asked Bernie to tell her more about his experience of her and of their work together. The supervisee said he felt that Carolyn was disinterested in him and in the supervised case; that she was "dead—bored and boring," and that her comments about his clinical work seemed perfunctory. Carolyn was surprised by Bernie's comments but realized with some discomfort that, in fact, she had experienced *his* work with his patient as affectively flat and sometimes boring. Not sure what to make of this, Carolyn said she would reflect on Bernie's remarks and that they would talk more about it next time.

In the next supervisory session, Carolyn told Bernie that she would like to discuss more fully what might be in play in the transference and countertransference between them, and between Bernie and his patient. She said that she thought that Bernie had detected something real, that she may not have been as engaged with his clinical work as he wanted her to be, or as she would like to be. Sharing that upon reflection, she recognized that they were having similar experiences of one another as dead, Carolyn asked Bernie if he had any ideas about what that could mean in terms of the supervised treatment or the supervision. For instance, was boredom and deadness "alive" in his work with the supervised patient?

Bernie reacted with fury, accusing Carolyn of trying to turn the tables on him and make the deadness his problem. Like so many teachers and supervisors before her, and like his previous analyst, she talked a good game about mutuality but really could not acknowledge what was, in fact, her own issue. When Carolyn stated that she actually thought Bernie's experience of her both accurately reflected her behavior with him *and* had potentially broader meaning for their relationship, and possibly for his work with his patient, Bernie once again accused Carolyn of begging the issue of her own lack of engagement.

In the following supervisory meeting, Bernie began by acknowledging that he had attacked unnecessarily and had distorted what Carolyn had said to him. He was beginning to realize that he had terminated his analysis before working through a very similar transference and countertransference matrix with his analyst. Reluctant to return to treatment for a variety of reasons, Bernie asked Carolyn if they could continue to address the "dead and boring thing" in supervision. Carolyn replied that she was willing to try to help Bernie work with this issue as it affected his relationship with her and his work with his patient.

Bernie told Carolyn that his mother was extremely ill for most of his childhood, often hovering near death, before finally succumbing to a rare blood disease when he was 13. Although she apparently tried to rally her strength during Bernie's daily visits to her sickroom, his mother's illness left her unable to show much interest in his activities, and Bernie often felt he was "boring her to death." At the same time, he was angry at her inability to engage with him and her apparently perfunctory remarks about the events in his life.

Even though Bernie could grasp intellectually the links between his relationship with his mother and his repetitive experience of important others in his life as dead or deadening, bored or boring, this insight did not seem to help him contain or manage his transference reactions to Carolyn. Over the next 6 weeks of supervision, he continued to struggle with rage at Carolyn for her lack of engagement, which he now perceived to be deliberate. Nothing Carolyn said succeeded in co-creating with Bernie a transitional space within the supervision where they could speak about his responses to her as material to be understood analytically.

After another 2 weeks of turbulent supervisory sessions, Carolyn told Bernie that she did not feel that their work was furthering resolution of his intense negative feelings about her and that, therefore, they were not able to attend adequately to his professional development. Carolyn said she felt that Bernie was an insightful and often wonderfully attuned clinician but that his functioning as both a clinician and a person in relationship with others would profit from additional analytic work. Bernie teared up and, weeping, begged Carolyn to continue to try to help him, because he had no where else to go. Moved, Carolyn responded that Bernie must have felt just that way in relationship to his mother but stated that the supervision could not provide him with what he needed and deserved to help him with something that was so clearly enormously painful for him. She said that she was willing to continue supervising Bernie, but they would have to focus more directly on his clinical work with the supervised patient than on his negative reactions to her, which she told him, would be pursued more fruitfully in treatment. Carolyn added that many clinicians, herself included, returned to analysis or therapy when unresolved psychological issues became salient and/or when a crisis occurred in their lives.

In the next supervisory session, Bernie looked drawn. He said he thought Carolyn had been very fair to him but that he wanted to terminate their supervision. He was not ready to return to therapy but was aware that the supervision was bogged down by his inability either to contain and manage or to make any real progress on his negative experience of Carolyn. Exhausted, Bernie planned to take a leave of absence from the program until he could decide what to do next. Carolyn, in turn, expressed her regret that she had not been able to find a way to create a supervisory space in which it was possible for him to engage in supervision primarily focused on his professional growth.

Here, Bernie and Carolyn were unable to co-construct a supervisory process that, while analytic, remained subservient to the supervisee's professional growth. The intensity of the relational matrix at play between them was too much for the supervision to hold and to address analytically, while primarily focusing on the supervisee's clinical work. Rather, the supervision was submerged in transference material that seemed to require further processing with a therapist, who could assist Bernie to work through his unresolved experiences with and conflicts about his dying mother.

When, on the other hand, the supervisee is not currently in treatment but has highly developed self-analytic capabilities, teaching and "treating" can be blurred more comfortably, with both parties secure in the knowledge that personal issues elucidated in supervision can be held and processed further in the supervisee's self-analysis. Here, the approach usually is akin to that experienced when the supervisee *is* in concurrent therapy or analysis. In rare instances, however, the supervisee who has completed his analysis may make temporary therapeutic use of the supervisor to address circumscribed psychodynamic material that interferes with his clinical work and is not wholly accessible to working through in self-analysis.

Although temporary therapeutic use of the supervisor falls under the rubric of the teach/treat boundary, the supervision literature is virtually silent on it as a specific possibility that deserves its own consideration. An exception is Robert Marshall (1993), whose supervisee took to the couch for 2 weeks to work through a temporary but disruptive crisis in her life. Harris and Ragen (1995), who engaged in mutual supervision that included mutual analysis of their countertransferences, offer a more egalitarian blurring of supervision and analysis. It is unlikely that many supervisory dyads can successfully contain a temporary shift to overt analysis without submerging their primary focus on the supervisee's professional development. Yet it is possible that, in certain situations, a circumscribed and short-lived excursion by supervisor and supervisee into a more explicitly therapeutic mode might be helpful and appropriate in advancing the supervisee's confidence and professional competence by working through a problematic countertransference or by restoring the trainee's optimal level of psychic functioning when, for some reason, it has been disrupted. An example from the experience of one of us (Frawley-O'Dea, 1998) expands on this point.

My (Frawley-O'Dea) final postdoctoral supervision began about 6 months after the termination of my analysis. Although the termination was a mutually agreed-on process, my analyst and I were aware of potentially unresolved issues regarding my response to envious maternal figures. We decided together, however, that this dynamic simply was not salient enough in my life at that point to warrant continued work.

About halfway through the yearlong supervision with a relationally oriented female analyst, the unresolved issues came alive with a vengeance when a female relative, with whom I had a long and complex history, launched an impressive, envious attack on an important celebration in my life. In the weeks following the event, I was quite regressed and withdrawn, a response that affected my work as well as most other domains of my functioning. As weeks turned into a month, I began to consider returning to treatment. At about that time, during one supervisory session, my supervisor asked me if I was OK, or something like that, indicating that she noticed that I was not the self she had come to know. Perhaps because my experience of this supervisor was of an exceptionally open, flexible woman, I, at first, quite tentatively, shared aspects of my history and my current crisis with this relative. She responded in a way that seemed to invite me to use her as I saw fit regarding this issue.

The following three supervisory meetings clearly were more therapy than supervision of case material. They were enormously helpful and initiated a working through, continued in self-analysis, of a longstanding and terribly painful internalized relational configuration that had come to life vividly at that time. After those sessions, we returned primarily to my patients, with occasional monitoring of how I was doing with the therapeutic issue in my self-analysis. At the end of the supervision, we discussed my temporary use of my supervisor as an analyst and, together, concluded that the working through of this aspect of my psychological organization had enriched the supervisory year for both of us. Furthermore, I have speculated since then that my reaction to intensely hateful envy from a woman might well have been worked through more powerfully with my female supervisor than it could have been with my male analyst.

What may be a very important element in this vignette is that I, the supervisee, although not currently in treatment, had completed a largely successful analysis. Moreover, a discrete life crisis evoked persecutory internal objects to which I was still partially in thrall and presented both the need and the opportunity for further, yet circumscribed, analytic work. Had I never been in treatment, had the need been for more pervasive structural change, or had the processing of this particular dynamic issue not proceeded with some speed, it is unlikely that supervision could have or should have been expected to provide analytic space sufficient to address fully enough an important personal dynamic, while preserving the overarching learning goals of the supervisory relationship. We are not suggesting, therefore, that supervision be considered a suitable, sole venue for protracted therapeutic work with a supervisee. Rather, we propose that within a relational model of teaching and "treating," supervisor and supervisee may, on probably quite rare occasions, agree to use the supervisory space temporarily to address a salient dynamic issue with a supervisee who has completed treatment, especially when that issue clearly is impeding the supervisory dyad's ability to focus well on the supervisee's clinical work and professional growth. In such a situation, the parameters of which are mutually delimited by the members of the supervisory dyad, use of the supervisor as analyst can further the goal of helping the supervisee develop as a psychoanalyst.

The "teach" component of the tripartite model of psychoanalytic training is most unambiguously located in the candidate's didactic courses. Similarly, the "treat" element of training is most clearly placed within the analytic relationship. Supervisor and supervisee, however, are entwined in at least two and, often, three relationships—analyst in training/supervisee and patient, supervisee and supervisor, supervisee/patient and analyst—that draw the supervisory dyad inexorably into an intricate relational web that, perforce, straddles the worlds of teaching and "treating." Neither rigid adherence to a taboo against "treating" in supervision nor a careless, anything-goes stance is optimal for the supervisee's continued personal and professional growth. Rather, careful, respectful, mutually determined construction of blurred teaching and "treating" uniquely suited to each supervisory dyad is most consistent with a model of supervision as a relationally mediated, analytic experience in and of itself.

CHAPTER 8

Parallel Process Revisited

Parallel process, which refers to the means by which the super-visory dyad enacts one or more key dynamics also alive in the treat-ment dyad, is another topic that has captured the imagination of a widely divergent group of analysts and has been repeatedly revisited in the psychoanalytic supervision literature (Arlow, 1963; Baudry, 1993; Caligor, 1984; Doehrman, 1976; Ekstein and Wallerstein, 1972; Frawley-O'Dea, 1997a; Gediman and Wolkenfeld, 1980; Grey and Fiscalini, 1987; Hirsch, 1997; Horner, 1988; Issacharoff, 1984; Jarmon, 1990; Lawner, 1989; Lester and Robertson, 1995; Marshall, 1997; Miller and Twomey, 1999; Rock, 1997; Rosiello, 1989; Sachs and Shapiro, 1976; Searles, 1955; Stimmel, 1995).

PARALLEL PROCESS: THE DEVELOPMENT OF A CONCEPT

Harold Searles (1955) is generally acknowledged as the first analyst to describe parallel process, although he himself used the term "reflection process." Searles and others after him (Arlow, 1963; Horner, 1988; Lawner, 1989; Sachs and Shapiro, 1976) view parallel process as an "up-ward bound" phenomenon. Specifically, the sources of parallel process are the patient and the therapeutic relationship. In these one-person, hierarchical models of parallel process, the concept of identification is paramount. The therapist is thought to identify unconsciously with some domain of the patient's psychological functioning. This may be resistance to certain material, an unconscious affective state, a self- or object representation, or a self-state currently out of awareness. Since the analyst is unaware of the identification, he cannot verbally discuss this aspect of the patient in supervision but, rather, enacts the patient's dynamic with the supervisor. For instance, a therapist may be working with a woman who cannot find words to describe her experience of her relationship growing up with her mother because it will evoke affects and representations of herself and her mother that are unbearably painful. In turn, the therapist may find himself similarly unable to speak to his supervisor about his experience of the patient, or himself in relationship with the patient. In this case, the therapist unconsciously has identified with his patient's resistance, expressed through wordlessness, perhaps in part because the patient's material is evocative for the therapist of his own maternal relationship.

In these constructions of parallel process, it is the role of the supervisor to maintain an observational stance. The supervisor, assumed to be the most self-aware member of the treatment and supervisory dyads, the most capable of detached observation, and the least emotionally involved in the supervised treatment, uses her reactions to the supervisee to elucidate the parallel process at work in the supervision. In the example of the wordless patient and therapist/supervisee used earlier, the supervisor would notice the therapist's difficulty in speaking about certain aspects of his clinical work, bring it to the supervisee's attention, and interpret it in terms of the supervisee's identification with the patient's psychological functioning.

This conceptualization of the unidirectionality and hierarchical discernment and interpretation of parallel process is consistent with one-person models of psychoanalytic treatment. Here, the source of the "problem" expressed through the parallel process is located within the patient in the analytic dyad, and within the supervisee in the supervisory dyad. At the same time that the problem—the anxiety, defense, resistance—is conveyed upward, knowledge about and interpretation of the salient psychological material are reflected downward from supervisor to supervisee/therapist to patient. This view does not have space for a discussion of parallel process as mutually constructed, enacted, observed, and interpreted by all the participants in the supervisory and therapeutic dyads. Nor is there room for an assignment of meaning to the material expressed in a parallel process that is negotiated between the patient and the analyst, or between the supervisee and the supervisor. In fact, Sachs and Shapiro (1976), discussing an example of parallel process, aver that "we could infer what was going on in the therapy by noticing *what the therapist was doing to us*" (p. 404, emphasis added).

As contemporary, two-person models of psychoanalytic treatment developed, the literature on parallel process shifted to include two-dyad, three-person paradigms of parallel process (Baudry, 1993; Buechler, 1996; Doehrman, 1976; Gediman and Wolkenfeld, 1980; Grey and Fiscalini, 1987; Jarmon, 1990; Marshall, 1997; Lester and Robertson, 1995; Stimmel, 1995), in which patient, therapist/supervisee, and supervisor actively participate in the creation and enactment of a parallel process. In these conceptualizations of parallel process, it is suggested that a parallel process can begin with the patient, supervisee, or supervisor; involve the other dyadic partner first in an intradyadic relational pattern; then, "carried" by the analyst/supervisee, influence the second dyad to enact a related transference–countertransference matrix. A parallel process is most likely to occur when the relational constellations carried from one dyad to the next fit the transference–countertransference predispositions of each dyad.

Both traditional and contemporary models of parallel process organize their views about the basis of parallel process around three themes: (1) identificatory processes leading to parallels between treatment and supervision, (2) transference and countertransference paradigms in one dyad that are enacted in parallel in the other, and (3) parallels *of* process that highlight the similarities between psychoanalysis and psychoanalytic supervision. In a relational model of parallel process, the first two themes overlap and reflect the transference–countertransference configuration at play in a given dyad.

Most psychoanalytic writers (Arlow, 1963; Baudry, 1993; Caligor, 1984; Gediman and Wolkenfeld, 1980; Horner, 1988; Issacharoff, 1984; Lawner, 1989) rely on some view of identificatory mechanisms (e.g., transient empathic identifications, treatment-threatening counter-identifications, projective identifications), to account for parallel processes. Issacharoff (1984), for example, adhering to an upward bound, one-person view of parallel process, proposes that parallel process results when the therapist temporarily and unconsciously identifies with some aspect of the patient's dynamic functioning and enacts that dynamic with the supervisor. The earlier example of the therapist who identifies with his patient's wordlessness is consistent with Issacharoff's view. Working from a contemporary, multidirectional, three-person paradigm of parallel process, on the other hand, Gediman and Wolkenfeld (1980) state that identifications can begin between any two dyadic partners—patient and therapist or supervisee and supervisor—and come to influence the relational patterns of both dyads. Here, for instance, a supervisor may be intimidated by her supervisee's ability to use humor in her clinical work. The supervisor unconsciously criticizes the supervisee's humorous remarks when they review audiotapes of the supervisee's work. Hurt by her supervisor's criticisms, which are reminiscent of her father's taciturn attitude toward human relations, the therapist unconsciously identifies with her supervisor's defense and begins to disengage from her patient's use of humor in the analytic setting. The patient ends up feeling bereft, hurt, and criticized, somewhat like the therapist/supervisee does in the supervisory relationship.

Other analysts (Grey and Fiscalini, 1987; Lester and Robertson, 1995; Stimmel, 1995) posit that parallel processes stem from transference and countertransference constellations at work either in the treatment or the supervision and parallel into the other dyad. For example, a patient may experience his male therapist as a persecutory, demanding father who is never pleased. The therapist who is uncomfortable with the patient's transference may not become consciously aware of it and therefore ignores the derivatives of the transference, for example, the patient's comment that "You probably won't think this is much of a dream but . . . " Rather than consciously working with the patient's transference, the therapist resists awareness of it and instead begins to experience the supervisor as a persecutory figure who never can be satisfied.

Finally, a number of writers (Baudry, 1993; Gediman and Wolkenfeld, 1987; Grey and Fiscalini, 1987) point to the procedural similarities of psychoanalysis and supervision, suggesting that parallel processes are predictable outcomes of these likenesses. Gediman and Wolkenfeld (1987) and Baudry (1993) even cite the same three structural similarities of supervision and psychoanalytic treatment to support the inevitability of parallel process: (1) Both are helping processes; (2) both require use of the self; and (3) both rely, at least in part, on multiple identificatory processes. These authors argue that the analytic and supervisory processes overlap and therefore invite regressive and progressive enactments of multidirectional parallelisms.

A RELATIONAL VIEW OF PARALLEL PROCESS

In this model, parallel process refers to the means by which key relational patterns of one dyad come to influence the relational configuration of the other dyad. Parallel processes are most likely to be set in motion when the transference–countertransference matrix in play in the first dyad involves nonverbal, unsymbolized relational constellations that are central to the relational functioning of that dyad but have not yet been consciously processed and linguistically encoded by the members of that dyad. Since these transference and countertransference phenomena are not consciously available to either member of the originating dyad, they cannot be talked about and worked through in that dyad. Rather, the first dyad becomes mired in an endless, uninterpreted enactment of one particular transference–countertransference mix. A parallel process enactment of a similar relational pattern offers members of the first dyad another chance to consciously access the meaning of their relationship by transferring elements of it to the second dyad, whose members may better be able to notice and name them. Parallel process is best understood, therefore, as an interdyadic transference–countertransference situation based on sequential enactment of identifications, often, projective identifications. While a parallel process can originate in either the treatment or the supervisory dyad, it is the supervisee who, by her overlapping membership in both dyads, necessarily is the interdyadic conduit of the relational material expressed through a parallel process.

Since parallel process relies on the enactment of transference and countertransference patterns often based on sequential projective identifications carried by the supervisee from one dyad to the next, we include in our elaboration of parallel process a relational paradigm of projective identification.

Projective Identification

Projective identification is a slippery notion that tends to be enshrouded in such an aura of mystery and the seemingly magical that some analysts reject the concept entirely (Stolorow, Orange, and Atwood, 1998). Other psychoanalytic writers have been captivated by the idea of projective identification and have developed and refined its meaning with passion (Bion, 1959, 1962; Grotstein, 1985; Kernberg, 1976, 1984; Klein, 1946; Ogden, 1982, 1986). Most conceptualizations of projective identification delineate two stages of the process: First, the patient projects a disowned aspect of her internalized relational world; second, the analyst identifies with the projection and, in addition, feels compelled to act in accordance with the contents of the projected material. We view projective identification as a particular kind of transference–countertransference phenomenon and find Davies and Frawley's (1994) comparison of projective identification to other levels of transference and counter-transference helpful in defining projective identification as a relational mechanism. Here, we extend their model of transference and counter-transference, and apply it to parallel process.

Davies and Frawley (1994) define one relational configuration or level of transference and countertransference as the conscious responses analyst and patient have toward one another. For example, a patient may tell her analyst that she feels like a little girl gently being rocked to sleep as she reclines on the analytic couch. In turn, the analyst is fully conscious of his maternal response to the patient and easily can imagine the scene described by his patient. Here is a transference and counter-transference matrix of which both parties are conscious and about which they are able to speak. In a parallel process enactment of this level of transference and countertransference, the analyst/supervisee may experience himself as securely held and nurtured by his supervisor. In turn, the supervisor is conscious of her protective, nurturing relational reaction to this supervisee. Since both supervisor and supervisee are conscious of this parallel, it can be discussed easily in supervision.

According to Davies and Frawley (1994), a second transference and countertransference situation encompasses transference or coun-tertransference reactions that are out of the patient's or analyst's awareness but are easily brought to consciousness through the analytic work. Here, a patient may sense that her male analyst is envious of an impressively large bonus she was awarded at work and fears that he will retaliate by withdrawing, or worse, by raising his fees. The analyst has not been conscious of his envy but recognizes it as soon as the patient brings it up. The analyst, however, does not feel compelled to express his envy through destructive retaliation but rather experiences himself somewhat like a proud father of a very successful daughter. When he says as much to the patient, the patient realizes that she had been dreading that her analyst would respond to her as her father so often had in the past. In this case, there is a transference and countertrans-ference constellation in play that easily is brought to the awareness of both members of the dyad.

A parallel process enactment of this type of transference and countertransference is also possible. Here, as the therapist discusses the clinical work with his supervisor, he becomes aware that he, like his patient, is concerned that the supervisor may be envious that he recently had a paper published in a prestigious journal. The supervisee tells the supervisor that, in talking about his patient, he realized that he, too, feared an envious response to an important accomplishment. Upon reflection, the supervisor recognizes that she, indeed, is envious that the supervisee has been published in a journal years earlier in his career than she was first published. Like the supervisee with his patient, however, the supervisor—now secure in her professional standing—does not feel the need to act out her envy in a destructive way. Having acknowledged her envy, she is freed to share warmly in her supervisee's success.

Finally, Davies and Frawley (1994) assert that at the level of projective identification, there are profoundly split off, powerful, nonverbal, unsymbolized transference and countertransference reactions that seem to grip the dyad and that temporarily immerse the analyst and patient in uninterpreted enactment. This is the level of transference and countertransference for which words are not available to the patient or the analyst. Rather, the analyst is likely to experience the relational configuration in play through nonverbal and inchoate countertransference experiences: affects, moods, somatic sensations, elusive images, and fantasies. This is the kind of transference–countertransference matrix that often is unconsciously transferred to the supervisory dyad by the supervisee in the unconscious hope of obtaining help in consciously elaborating and putting words to the relational patterns now being enacted in both dyads. The following case illustrates projective identification in the clinical setting that is expressed through a parallel process enactment in the supervisory dyad. It illustrates how important a supervisor can be in helping a supervisee come to consciousness about and, then, more effectively manage a previously profoundly unconscious relational enactment at play in the treatment dyad.

Jerry, an experienced analyst, found himself literally falling asleep during sessions with Melanie, a woman whose parents had bound and beaten her as a child. Melanie, who had hazy memories of these experiences, reported them to Jerry with an incongruent, upbeat affect. Despite Melanie's seemingly engaging presentation, and no matter what Jerry would do to stay awake—open a window, drink a cup of coffee prior to the session, splash cold water in his face before meeting the patient—within fifteen minutes of Melanie's arrival, Jerry's eyes would droop as sleep overtook him. His subjective experience at these times was of complete powerlessness and he found himself vaguely picturing Dorothy in *The Wizard of Oz* as she fell under the influence of the poppies.

Melanie used the couch and seemed not to notice Jerry's naps. Rather, she consciously experienced him as concerned and caring. Eventually, Jerry came to understand his sleep as an introjective iden-tification with a self-state of Melanie's that had once helped her cope with her parents' abuse and now represented a defense against fully reexperiencing her relationship with them. Melanie once offhandedly described feeling as though she had lived most of her life in a dense fog, barely able to see her way through the mists enveloping her. She unconsciously was terrified of entering that fog in treatment, instead maintaining a focused and even perky persona. It was only when Jerry, through an introjective identification with Melanie's disowned self-state-in-the-fog, entered, survived, and gradually gave words to the fog that it became detoxified enough for Melanie to experience it again herself in Jerry's presence. This occurred with the help of Jerry's super-visor.

In supervision with Ted, Jerry described his bouts of sleep but he did so in a lively way, even laughing about those episodes. He had no access in supervision to the feelings of sleepiness that assailed and engulfed him during the clinical sessions. Ted, however, began to feel uncharacteristi-cally bored with Jerry's presentation of his patient and found himself drifting off, thinking of other things. Ted also had trouble remembering or caring about what Jerry had to say about Melanie. When Ted tried to formulate something about the supervised treatment or about the super-visory relationship, he felt sluggish and unwilling to focus attentively enough to formulate thoughts and then put them into words.

The parallel supervisory transference and countertransference process went on for several weeks, until Jerry verbalized noticing that he could not capture the drowsy state he experienced during his ses-sions with Melanie when he presented them in supervision. At that point, Ted became able to describe his recent experience of the super-vision and to suggest that it might be connected to the relational ma-trix in play in the supervised treatment. The relational impasse in su-pervision was broken. Jerry and his supervisor began to describe verbally what had been happening between them. They then hypoth-esized that Melanie's perky, focused, confident self-structure coexisted with another "fogged-out" organization of self, a self-structure that re-mained detached from her abusive experiences and the pain they could evoke for her. It was at this point that Jerry became able to stay awake with Melanie and to talk with her about the transference and countertransference at work between them. Here, Jerry transferred back to the treatment a parallel version of the supervisory dyad's ability to use words to consciously elaborate, think about, and verbally discuss a relational configuration important to the treatment dyad.

As this vignette suggests, one important function of a projective identification is that it provides an opportunity for one member of a dyad to experience, contain, process, and put words to an experience of self or other that is central to the internal relational world of the other member of the dyad but currently split off from the conscious awareness of that person and, therefore, not available for verbal discussion.

The psychoanalytic literature has addressed the ways in which an analyst can optimally handle projective identifications as they arise in the clinical setting. Notions such as "holding" (Winnicott, 1947), "metabolizing," and "containing" (Bion, 1959, 1962; Ogden, 1982, 1994) all have been developed as vital to the analyst's successful processing of a projective identification originating with the patient. Each of these paradigms present the analyst more or less as an empty vessel, ready and waiting to be filled up with the patient's projective material. A relational model of holding and projective identification (Slochower, 1996), however, suggests instead that the analyst comes to his clinical work with his own subjectivity and his own psychodynamics. A given analyst, therefore, will be predisposed to take on certain projective identificatory experiences rather than others. In addition, he will enact the projective identification in a way that is influenced by his own psychological functioning. In the example of Jerry's work with Melanie, the analyst enacted the patient's split-off-in-the-fog self-structure by falling asleep. Another analyst might not be susceptible to that particular projective identification at all or might engage with it differently, perhaps by daydreaming or unconsciously ending the session early.

Like projective identification, parallel process is a relationally mediated phenomenon, the usual function of which is to allow one dyad to assist the other in containing, enacting, noticing, reflecting on, processing, and, ultimately, putting words to important but unformulated transference and countertransference material operating in the first dyad. Also, like the analyst working with a projective identificatory process, a supervisor will engage through her own subjectivity with a supervisee's introduction into the supervisory space of a relational striving parallel to one operating in the supervised treatment. Supervisors, depending on their unique psychological organizations, will be more available to the enactment of certain parallel process transference–countertransference matrices than to others. In addition, they will respond to the supervisee in keeping with their own psychodynamic functioning. In the vignette involving Jerry and Ted, for instance, the supervisor did not react to Jerry by falling asleep, as Jerry did with Melanie. However, the supervisor's disinterest, distractedness, and sluggishness closely enough replicated Jerry's countertransferential identification with Melanie's in-the-fog organization of self that supervisor and supervisee were able to connect it to the supervised treatment.

Neuroscientific Constructions of Projective Identification and Parallel Process

All psychoanalytic constructions of projective identification and of parallel process attempt to encode linguistically what are essentially nonverbal relational interactions. In addition, the interpersonally mediated processes resulting in any identifications, especially projective identifications, as well as those expressed through parallel processes, are poorly understood. Recent neuroscientific thinking, however, is beginning to demystify the concepts of projective identification and parallel process by providing plausible neurobiological explanations for these phenomena. Panskepp (1999), for instance, postulates that there are at least two domains of consciousness and unconsciousness—cognitive and affective—involving different brain pathways. The cognitive continuum of consciousness to unconsciousness is cortically mediated and linguistically represented. In this system of consciousness–unconsciousness, unconscious material probably was once known to the patient, symbolically represented, and then repressed. On the other hand, the affective range of consciousness to unconsciousness is nonrepresentational and mediated by subcortical parts of the brain. It is likely that unconscious material in this system was never cognitively known to the patient and never linguistically encoded and then repressed. Rather, it is possible that the affective unconscious represents dissociated material that is available primarily as affects, body states, or moods.

Panskepp's (1999) nascent model potentially offers a neurobiological paradigm for projective identification and for parallel process, both of which are often first experienced by the analyst or supervisor as wordless, formless, somatic/affective subjective states. Perhaps, while the therapist and the patient, and the supervisee or supervisor, are engaged in cortically mediated, primarily linguistically represented conversation, they simultaneously relate unconsciously through a subcortically driven, wordless attunement to dissociated, primarily affectively and somatically experienced states. This view of projective identification and of parallel process supports the traditionally expressed need for the therapist or supervisor to take in, tolerate, and "metabolize" the projective identification (Grotstein, 1985; Ogden, 1982; Tansey and Burke, 1989) exemplified in Jerry's sleepiness with Melanie, or in his supervisor's sluggishness with him. What this may in fact mean neurobiologically is that the analyst or supervisor begins to engage with the projective identificatory or parallel process experience cortically, linguistically representing it for what might be the first time, and then gradually helps the patient or supervisee to put words to his own similar internal experience.

PARALLEL PROCESS IN EVERYDAY LIFE

Like the concept of projective identification, the idea of parallel process as developed in the supervision literature has been either idealized or devalued for its apparent status as a mysterious and mystifying process unique to psychoanalytic work. We, however, agree with the view espoused by Grey and Fiscalini (1987) that parallel processes, like transference and countertransference matrices and identifications, including projective ones, are basic components of relational life traversing all interpersonal settings.

A familiar extratherapeutic example of everyday parallel process is the "kick the dog" phenomenon. Here, a businessman, anxious to please his boss, verbally is torn to shreds by that boss over an apparently minor mistake. Unable to retaliate, and forced by the work situation to humbly suffer his boss's ire, the businessman simmers with unexpressed rage and humiliation all day. That night, when his vulnerable and anxious-to-please 4-year-old son old greets him wearing dad's best shirt, now adorned with Play-Doh, the businessman verbally berates the child until he slinks away in humiliation. The businessman may not be conscious of the connection between his day at work, his identification with his boss, his projection onto his son of his devalued self-representation, and the excessiveness of his reaction to his son. However, this is parallel process, alive and well, being played out in everyday life.

Grey and Fiscalini (1987), like most psychoanalytic writers, focus on "negative" parallel process. Positively mediated parallel processes also are found in normal human relations. For example, 6-year-old Pete is jealous and angry when his 3-year-old sister is doted on after her somewhat complicated appendectomy. He is sullen, withdrawn, and nasty to his sister. Pete's first-grade teacher, Jane Kelley, notices a change in his school behavior, speaks with his mom about the situation at home, and spends some extra time working with him individually on an art project he enjoys. After a few weeks of this, Pete's behavior toward his sister softens, and he even teaches her how to draw a dinosaur like the one he has worked on with his teacher. Once again, parallel process is seen in everyday relational workings of life, this time from a positive, healing parallel of Pete's relationship with his teacher into an improved relationship with his sister. Here, Pete identifies with Jane Kelley's compassionate stance and applies it toward his sister.

The multidirectionality of parallel process also plays out in this scenario. Jane Kelley's younger sister is in the midst of planning a big wedding, whereas there are no romantic prospects on the horizon for Jane. Without fully realizing it, Jane, filled with envy toward her younger sister, has been demeaning and sarcastic with her recently. Jane's talk with Pete's mom and her work with Pete unconsciously affect Jane, leading her to be more supportive and celebratory of her sister.

These vignettes suggest that, while it is important for clinicians to have a theoretical understanding of parallel process, it also is helpful to grasp its ubiquity in human relations. Such demystification of parallel process may render its exploration in supervision less precious and more accessible as an ordinary relational mechanism, one that can originate in any dyad, parallel into the other, and reverberate back and forth for some time.

While parallel process may be operative in many human relations in which two dyads or groups share at least one common member, the procedural or structural similarities of psychodynamic treatment and supervision—the parallels *of* process mentioned by other writers (Baudry, 1993; Gediman and Wolkenfeld, 1980; Grey and Fiscalini, 1987)— heighten the possibility that one way in which the supervisory and

treatment dyads will influence each other is through parallel enactment of transference and countertransference experiences, some of
which are based on projective identification. Adding complexity to a
relational model of parallel process is an understanding that parallel
process does not always connote identical process. In other words, although the treatment and supervisory dyads may enact a similar relational pattern, sometimes they will engage in relational processes that
are dissimilar but interrelated. In this case, one dyad plays out a relational configuration currently dissociated from but central to the relational life of the other dyad. Here, we use "symmetrical parallel
process" to denote the enactment of similar transference and countertransference constellations in both dyads. When, on the other hand,
one dyad enacts a split-off facet of an important relational matrix *not*
currently operative in the other dyad, we term this "asymmetrical parallel process." In what follows, we focus on the third level of parallel
process described earlier: parallel processes that are out of the conscious awareness of patient, analyst/supervisee, and supervisor. These,
the most difficult parallels to identify and to put into words, are the focus of the rest of this chapter. We look first at symmetrical parallel
process.

Symmetrical Parallel Process

Symmetrical parallel process is the kind of parallel process most often
cited in the supervision literature and illustrated so far in this chapter.
The central conceptualization of symmetrical parallel process is that a
transference and countertransference configuration arises in either the
supervised treatment or in the supervision. At this point, the relational pattern in play is out of the conscious awareness of the members of
the dyad. It is not available for conscious elaboration, discussion,
meaning making, or negotiation because it has not been linguistically
formulated yet by either party to the dyad. The supervisee, however,
the common member of both dyads, nonverbally exerts relational
pressure on the member of the other dyad to enact a similar transference and countertransference matrix with the supervisee, in the often
unconscious hope that someone can contain, enact, process, and put
words to what is transpiring now in both dyads. The key to symmetrical parallel process is that both the treatment and the supervisory
dyads play out similar relational constellations.

Symmetrical parallel process can express at least two transference and countertransference paradigms. In the first, the patient and the therapist identify with and enact reciprocal aspects of the patient's internal world, the latter usually through projective identification. Specifically, one identifies with a self-representation and the other with an object representation, in a relational matrix somewhat akin to Racker's (1968) concept of complementary transference and countertransference. In turn, within the supervisory dyad, the supervisee and the supervisor also live out these reciprocal relational roles. Reciprocal transference and countertransference constellations can be organized around primitive, disturbing experiences of self and other (e.g., victim and victimizer), or can express more pleasant, satisfying relational themes (e.g., nurtured and nurturing). An example of symmetrical parallel process involving intensely disorganizing reciprocal relational constellations in both treatment and supervision illustrates this form of parallel process.

Catherine, an analytic candidate, brought to supervision her work with Janine, a 29-year-old woman with a history of childhood sexual and physical abuse, adolescent rape, and two adult relationships in which she had been battered. Janine was severely dissociative, affectively flat, and tended to relate to others in a formulaic victim–victimizer way. If she could not dominate the other, she expected only to be utterly and cruelly dominated.

When Janine began psychoanalytic psychotherapy with Catherine, she expressed how much she wanted to work hard in therapy to change her life. She never missed any of her twice-weekly sessions but the therapy sessions gradually began to feel torturous to both Catherine and her patient. A predictable pattern developed; Janine opened the session with a few stilted remarks but then seemed to freeze. She became almost mute, staring at Catherine with a look that conveyed both terror and a warning not to touch her. Catherine, too, felt herself to be muted and paralyzed. She wanted to help Janine, to find a way to reach her—to "touch" her analytically—but found herself unable to form too many words. She could not find it in herself to interpret or to ask about Janine's terror, in part because she felt so controlled by her patient's unyielding gaze. As they sat in ever more intolerable silence or exchanged a few forced words, Catherine began to despair that the treatment could progress. She dreaded the sessions but also felt inadequate and guilty about so utterly failing her patient.

After Catherine's initial presentation of Janine to Barbara, her supervisor, which was full of affect and vivid descriptions of the sessions and Catherine's countertransference experiences, the supervisory work began to parallel the therapeutic relationship. Catherine had come to supervision following an unpleasant prior supervisory year in which she felt "beat up" by her supervisor. In presenting Janine, Catherine also shared that she, too, had been physically abused as a child, although she did not feel that her traumatic history was at all as horrific as Janine's. Barbara also had childhood trauma in her history, having witnessed her father regularly beating her older brother. Like Catherine with Janine, Barbara hoped to help Catherine, both by contributing to her growth as a psychoanalyst and by repairing the wounds apparently inflicted by the previous supervisor. It is possible that, unconsciously, Barbara also wanted to heal Catherine's childhood scars as well as her own, now projected onto her supervisee. Yet as the weeks went by, Catherine and Barbara seemed stuck. It became increasingly difficult for Catherine to find words to describe her sessions with Janine, and her affect flattened. Catherine began to look fearful during the supervisory hours. In turn, Barbara felt more and more uncomfortable about herself during supervision with Catherine. She was afraid of hurting Catherine by pushing her to express more about the sessions with Janine, while, at the same time, she increasingly resented Catherine for the awkwardness of the supervisory time together. Like Catherine with her patient, Barbara also felt guilty about her failure to help her supervisee.

In this vignette, Catherine and the supervisor enacted a symmetrical parallel process constituted by similar, reciprocal transference and countertransference constellations. In each dyad, one person—Janine in treatment, Catherine in supervision—subjectively experienced herself as wanting and needing help. At the same time, both feared that the helper would damage her and therefore kept her at bay. Split off from conscious awareness, however, was another organization of self, identified with the aggressor, which was determined to stave off any "touch" or vulnerability by utterly controlling the relational scene. Catherine, as therapist, and Barbara, as supervisor, experienced themselves simultaneously as powerfully destructive and powerfully destroyed as analytic entities.

In this case, it was the patient who began to loosen the impasse at work in both dyads. Arriving at the session one day, Janine told Catherine that she did not think Catherine liked her very much. Catherine recognized for the first time how angry she was at Janine's unconscious attempts to control the sessions and the analyst's mind through her mute but unyielding stare.

In supervision, Catherine talked with renewed animation about her session with Janine. Barbara suggested to her that they had enacted a similar relational configuration in their own work, saying that, like Janine, Catherine might be worried about Barbara's feelings toward her and acknowledged that, like Catherine in her work with Janine, Barbara had felt both angry toward Catherine and guilty about not helping her. In turn, Catherine told Barbara that she was afraid the supervisor would think she was a failure as an analyst but, at the same time, she was angry that Barbara was not helping her much with her patient. Catherine and Barbara then began to talk more fully about their own relationship as it had developed so far, and the mutual influence of the supervision and the supervised treatment on what had occurred in each dyad.

As the supervision went on, Catherine and Barbara were able to use their understanding of this parallel process to represent symbolically aspects of Janine's experience of self and other that heretofore had been out of Janine's awareness and available to the therapeutic work only through enactment. This included Janine's aggressive determination to render the other powerless, while subjectively experiencing only her neediness and yearning to be helped. They also became increasingly freer to discuss the vicissitudes of their own relationship and its ongoing connection with the supervised treatment.

In this example of symmetrical parallel process, both the supervisory and treatment dyads enacted similar reciprocal transference and countertransference paradigms that reinforced each other. Catherine's increasing difficulty in the analytic relationship intensified the supervisory enactment and vice versa. When members of both dyads began to speak about what was happening between them in the respective and overlapping transference–countertransference situations, the progressive effect of more completely and symbolically representing the myriad affects, experiences, and fantasies about self and other, and even somatic states evoked in each member of the supervisory and treatment dyads, also reverberated between each dyad. Although the transference and countertransference configuration described here appeared and reappeared in both the treatment and the supervision, it did not become as immutable again. In addition, the discernment and discussion of this parallel process enactment within supervision allowed Catherine to reestablish analytic neutrality as defined in this model; she and her patient no longer were bogged down in an endless repetition of one relational pattern. Similarly, supervisory neutrality was restored; Catherine and Barbara were able to respond to one another with greater flexibility and openness.

It is clear that, in this vignette, there were individual characteristics of this patient, therapist/supervisee, and supervisor that may have predisposed them to get stuck more in this particular parallel process than in others. Each woman had a history of childhood trauma that may have made her more available to the enactment of certain relational paradigms than to others. Furthermore, one could speculate that, as former victims, each may have been especially uncomfortable with aggressive, controlling self-representations suggesting an identification with the aggressor.

Some analysts (Fosshage, 1997; Hirsch, 1997; Miller and Twomey, 1999) caution that analysts should be careful about assuming that a parallel process is at work, just because both dyads enact similar transference and countertransference constellations. They assert that independently derived yet similar relational paradigms may arise coincidentally in each dyad. Here, for example, the supervisory dynamic could stem as much from Catherine's own transference to the supervisor as a potentially helpful but equally dangerous object, and Barbara's countertransference experience of feeling simultaneously destructive and destroyed, as it could from Catherine's identification with Janine and the subsequent parallel process enactment of that identification.

In a somewhat different vein, Stimmel (1995) warns that the supervisor may use a parallel process metaphor to avoid knowing about and working through her relational responses toward the supervisee that represent her own transference or countertransference to the supervisee and have little to do with the patient. In the supervisory situation described here, for instance, Barbara's own internalized sense of herself as a victim, as well as a dissociated identification with her brutal father, could engender a transference to Catherine as a disruptive reminder of her own painful childhood and its sequelae for Barbara.

These writers raise important points. Overzealous invocation of parallel process to explain similar but coincidentally arising relational patterns in the treatment and supervisory dyads can obscure rather than clarify meaning. Any concept can be used defensively to ward off disturbing relational material. At the same time, overzealous rejection of parallel process ignores the psychoanalytic and neuroscientific literature supporting the possibility that this process influences in mean-ingful ways the relational patterns of two related dyads. The relational model of supervision proposed here encourages supervisor and super-visee to explore multiple levels of potential meaning in the transfer-ence and countertransference emerging in their work, one level of which may be the emergence of a parallel process. A relational shift may appear to be primarily located in the transference and counter-transference of the supervision but, when discussed by supervisor and supervisee, may seem to them to be related to the treatment as well. Or not. Almost always, a parallel process will also express an impor-tant aspect of the supervisory relationship itself, as that context must provide fertile ground for the parallel process to take root.

Janine, Catherine, and Barbara enacted a symmetrical parallel process involving similar reciprocal transference and countertransfer-ence paradigms at play in each dyad. Symmetrical parallel processes may also reflect congruent transference and countertransference con-figurations, a concept drawing on Racker's (1968) concordant trans-ference and countertransference. In a congruent relational paradigm, the analyst identifies with and experiences a self-representation of the patient, usually one that the patient is unaware of, or at least has not verbalized within the treatment. When a congruent transference and countertransference constellation is embodied in a parallel pro-cess, the supervisee unconsciously enacts his identification with the patient's self-representation with the supervisor. Here, the supervisor also identifies and experiences herself congruently with that organi-zation of self. An example of symmetrical parallel process involving congruent transference–countertransference matrices, evolving with-in treatment and supervisory dyads and primarily focused on living out reciprocal relational paradigms, illustrates this kind of parallel process.

Steve, a 19-year-old man and an only child, began twice-weekly psychoanalytic psychotherapy with Donna, a third-year doctoral candi-date. A central issue for Steve was his mother's death after a long ill-ness when he was 9 years old. His mother had been so sick for so long that he had only vague but warm memories of her loving presence when he was very young. After his mother's death, his father spent most of his time away from home. Steve was cared for primarily by his paternal grandmother, who was warm, nurturing, and playful. Unfor-tunately, this woman died about a year before Steve entered treatment. When he began therapy, Steve said he was functioning quite well and was generally "happy" but noticed that he had "no real goals or interests." He quickly formed an initial transference to Donna as a warm, caring replacement for his dead mother and grandmother.

Donna, 34 years old, was the second of four children. She felt very close to her older sister and two younger brothers, the youngest of whom was 20 and particularly special to Donna. Donna had a warm relationship with her mother, whom she perceived to have balanced a successful career with attentive mothering. She was less sure of her relationship with her father, a busy surgeon, whom she often experienced as both physically and emotionally unavailable. Donna's father passed away shortly before she began her training and her psychoanalysis; she felt he had died before she had the opportunity to address her relationship with him directly.

Donna chose Paul, her supervisor, in part because she had found him to be intelligent, funny, and open. Like her father, Paul could "cut to the core of a problem" but was also emotionally generous to his students. She quickly formed a transference to Paul as a generous, playful analytic father figure, in some ways a replacement for her intellectually gifted but forbidding and now dead father.

Paul, 56, was accurately perceived by Donna as intellectually excited about psychoanalytic ideas and clinical work. He enjoyed supervising students and derived a great deal of satisfaction from their professional growth. He also enjoyed the idealization he knew he evoked in students but did not need to preserve their idealizations at the expense of the supervisory work. He could be challenging and could tolerate being perceived as disappointing. A productive teacher, writer, and supervisor, with a wife and three children, Paul sometimes overextended and exhausted himself, at which times he could become withdrawn and distracted. The supervisory year with Donna was demanding both professionally and personally, with a book deadline and his son's Bar Mitzvah coinciding about midway through the supervision.

Both dyads began the supervisory year with similar, reciprocal transference and countertransference configurations in play. In the treatment, Donna felt very maternal toward Steve and enjoyed feeding him as much as he enjoyed being fed through the therapy. Similarly, Donna found Paul to be all that she hoped for and, in turn, Paul experienced Donna as a bright, dedicated student whose sense of humor meshed with his own.

This kind of symmetrical parallel process often goes unnoticed in supervision or is accepted without much further examination as a good working alliance in both the treatment and the supervision. As both Rock (1997) and Epstein (1997) point out, obvious problems in either the treatment or the supervision are likely to receive quicker and more intense supervisory focus than apparent smooth sailing. Periods of "unobjectionable" positive, symmetrical parallel process deserve to be noted and discussed by supervisor and supervisee lest they later become part of a defensive constellation obscuring other important transference–countertransference paradigms in the supervisory or treatment dyads. In this case, it was the enactment of a congruent parallel process that alerted the supervisory dyad to other relational themes at play in both settings.

During several sessions with Steve, Donna found herself feeling inexplicably sad and mournful, and fleeting images of her father passed through her mind. In discussing these sessions with Paul, she once again felt very sad but said nothing about this to her supervisor. Over the next few supervisory sessions, Paul also found himself feeling grief-stricken, with thoughts of his son arising as he spoke with Donna. Not sure what his feelings were about, Paul did not bring them up with her. Several weeks later, however, Donna finally described her feelings of sadness during her work with Steve. Paul asked her if she had experienced similar emotions in the supervisory sessions, and she acknowledged that she had. At that point, Paul told Donna about his own feelings of sadness and his associations to his recently "bar mitzvahed" son.

As the supervisory dyad discussed the sadness experienced by Donna in both dyads and by Paul in the supervisory setting, they realized that their individual grief feelings were associated with fantasies about impending loss. The supervisor became aware that the Bar Mitzvah of his youngest son represented for him the beginning of that child's more profound emotional and actual separation and that, in just a few years, there would be no children at home. Paul was not sure that he was ready for that developmental shift in his own life and feared that it might occur before he was psychologically prepared for it. In the supervisory dyad, Donna's sadness was related to her foreboding about the end of the supervisory year. Symbolically finding in Paul the father she never had, she was distraught that their relationship would end before she was emotionally willing to "leave home." In the therapeutic work with Steve, Donna associated her sadness with her sense of not having had enough time to work out her relationship with her father before he died.

As Donna and Paul discussed these experiences, they began to wonder if Steve was also unconsciously mournful about the possibility that his therapeutic relationship with Donna would end before he had worked through his need for her. When Donna asked Steve about this, he began to cry. Far from being an unconscious experience, Steve had been filled with a dreadful sadness in and out of the therapy sessions. He was sure that Donna would leave him long before he felt able to let go of her, and he already was grieving what seemed to be an unbearable upcoming loss. The patient had been unwilling to speak to Donna about his dread because he did not want to cry in front of her; weeping would cause him to feel even closer to her and more needy. In addition, he was reluctant to interfere with the warm, nurturing relational paradigm he was enjoying in the treatment by bringing up "negative" feelings.

It was Paul's and Donna's enactment, identification, and verbal processing of the parallel process of being filled with sadness that allowed each dyad to reach beyond the warm and satisfying reciprocal transference and countertransference configurations at play in a way that expanded and deepened the relationships both in supervision and in the supervised treatment.

Asymmetrical Parallel Process

Parallel processes also can be asymmetrical. In an asymmetrical parallel process, one dyad enacts a particular transference–countertransference configuration, while the other enacts a relational paradigm that is important to the first dyad but that currently is not being enacted in that dyad. Often, the relational matrix enacted in the second dyad is distinctly contradictory to the one that is in play in the first dyad. It is a relational pattern that bespeaks the centrality of a transference–countertransference mix currently dissociated from the first dyad, usually from the treatment situation. Indeed, it can be thought of as a postcard from the edge of the analytic relational scene advertising coming transference and countertransference events.

An asymmetrical parallel process may not even appear to be parallel process except that, upon further examination, usually by supervisor and supervisee, it becomes clear that the supervisory dyad is enacting a missing piece of the transference–countertransference situation of the treatment dyad. It is here that contemporary concepts of pathologically dissociated organizations of self may help elucidate an asymmetrical parallel process.

While asymmetrical parallel processes may characterize the work of any pair of supervisory and treatment dyads, they are likely to be particularly prominent when the supervised patient's history and character are marked by chaos, disorganization, trauma, or pronounced dissociative barriers between self-states. If there is some analog between the intensity of the analytic relational field and the relational configurations emerging in supervision, asymmetrical parallel processes will be most evident when the supervised treatment involves a more disturbed or dissociated patient. Furthermore, the relational complexities of a parallel process may deepen across the triad if supervisee and/or supervisor also have histories, organizations of self, or dissociative tendencies similar to the patient's.

Dissociation is the hallmark of trauma. It is a process of severing connections events between that seem irreconcilably different, events and their affective significance, events and cognitive awareness of their meaning, or events and their symbolic representation. Unlike repression, which is a horizontal division of conscious and unconscious mental contents, dissociation involves a vertical split of the ego that results in two or more self-states that are more or less organized and independently functioning. Such dissociative states are unavailable to the rest of the personality and, therefore, are not subject to psychic operations of elaboration. Rather, they are likely to make their presence known to the dissociated individual via the emergence of recurrent intrusive images, violent or symbolic enactments, inexplicable somatic sensations, repetitive nightmares, and psychosomatic conditions.

The analyst working with a patient for whom dissociation is a primary psychic mechanism is immersed in rapidly shifting, often wildly chaotic transference and countertransference paradigms. For protracted periods of time, much that occurs in the consultation room is nonverbally enacted through projective identificatory processes rather than being verbally represented. It often happens, therefore, that, like the patient, the analyst working with a dissociative patient is subjected to dissociative experiences himself, especially if he also has a personal history of trauma. During these periods of projected identification with a dissociated self-state or object representation of the patient, the therapist's symbolic capacities are submerged in inchoate fantasies, feelings, and sensorimotor sensations. Because clinical work with highly dissociative patients is fraught with very intense and rapidly shifting transference–countertransference mixes, it can happen that the treatment dyad becomes unable to hold, much less consciously process, all the relational configurations that are important to it. An asymmetrical parallel process offers the treatment dyad the opportunity to temporarily "store" a currently dissociated relational constellation in another dyad, until there is room for it in the clinical work. If supervisor and supervisee are able to notice, process, and put words to the relational patterns encompassed by an asymmetrical parallel process, the analyst/supervisee may be more capable of effectively handling the analogous transference–countertransference paradigm when it arrives on the analytic relational scene. An example makes this point.

Elsewhere, one of us (Frawley-O'Dea, 1997a) described her work with Christina, an adult who, as a child, was brutally sexually, physically, and emotionally tortured by her mother. The mother herself had utterly paradoxical manifestations of self. On the one hand, she was an active mother who took Christina to ballet lessons, cooked gourmet meals, led her daughter's Brownie troop, and volunteered at church. On the other hand, this mother sadistically penetrated Christina's anus with a dildo, kicked her around the room, and verbally tormented her. At still other times, Christina's mother sat for hours, mutely rocking in a chair in the family room, a remote and unavailable figure.

Perhaps not at all surprisingly, Christina developed her own quite paradoxically organized self-states, each forged in relationship with mindbendingly disparate aspects of her mother. One version of Christina was a bright, verbal, gregarious, high-functioning professional. Another was a chaotically organized woman who drank too much, stole, mutilated her body, and characteristically entered sexual relationships with married or abusive men. Boundary transgressions and unfettered impulse were at the core of this organization of Christina's personality. Like her mother, Christina also had a self that was depressed, withdrawn, barely connected to life.

In Christina's case, her various organizations of self were not the normative, healthy "distributions of the self into multiple islands of memory, affect, meaning, awareness, and intention" but rather represented, "the dissociation of the self into multiple subselves marooned on unbridgeable islands . . . the condition of a damage self" (Pizer, 1996, p. 504). Not only was Christina besieged by unbearably painful memories, fantasy elaborations, affects, and body states associated with her childhood experiences, but also their compartmentalization into totally incompatible behaviors, values, reactions to others, motivations, and ambitions—in short, vastly disparate self-states—left her feeling fragmented, literally out of self-control, on the edge of insanity.

About 6 months after I (Frawley-O'Dea) began working with Christina, I presented her in supervision. My former supervisor and I have written about our work on this case (Frawley-O'Dea, 1997a; Hirsch, 1997). Here, I focus on a particular asymmetrical parallel process in which a missing piece of the transference–countertransference configuration of the treatment was contained by and enacted in the supervisory relationship.

From the beginning of Christina's analysis, until I stopped presenting her in supervision, the analytic relationship was devoid of transference and countertransference paradigms related to the patient's attachment to or identification with either the hot, abusive mother or the frozen, almost catatonic mother. Rather, Christina and I engaged easily and playfully. The primary transference to me seemed to be as her father, with whom, as a little girl, she comfortably and securely twirled around the living room, dancing with her feet on his. In turn, I enjoyed her shy idealization of me and felt protective of her. Although we both acknowledged intellectually that our relationship would not stay so carefree forever, we seemed determined to preserve for the time being the mutually affectionate relational configuration currently in play.

During the months that I presented Christina in supervision, my supervisor and I were not having such an easy time of it. Despite my enthusiasm about working with him, we could not seem to find a comfortable way to work together. We understood the case from different theoretical perspectives and appeared to disagree fundamentally about treatment approaches. As the weeks went by, I felt increasingly anxious about each supervisory session, until the anxiety reached a paralyzing level. I was frozen, perhaps in a way somewhat analogous to how Christina felt with her frighteningly aroused, abusive mother. At the same time, I was more and more disappointed in and angry with my supervisor for what I perceived as his failure to help me with Christina. Finally, I found a way to present another patient to my supervisor. Almost immediately, I felt more at ease in supervision and experienced my supervisor as enormously helpful with the second patient.

Interestingly, almost as soon as I stopped discussing Christina in supervision, the transference–countertransference paradigm enacted between us shifted dramatically. Specifically, the violently abusive mother and one rendition of the frozen, confused child entered the analytic work. Christina, subjectively experiencing herself as my victim, in fact, enacted identification with her mother's vicious devaluation of her, vituperatively castigating me for weeks as being self-involved, amazingly inept, and wanting to humiliate her by having her need me. In turn, I countertransferentially identified with Christina as a child. I was shocked and frozen but believed that I must have been responsible for somehow turning my previously delighted and delightful patient into a crazy woman.

Unfortunately, my supervisor and I spent little time talking about the development of our own relationship until the end of the supervisory year. Nor did we actively wonder about what, if any, parallel processes might be coloring the analytic and supervisory spaces. Moreover, there were elements of the supervision itself that contributed to the frozenness between my supervisor and me. In retrospect, however, it seems very possible that an asymmetrical parallel process also was in operation, through which the frozenness of the transference–countertransference paradigm enacted by me and my supervisor represented and contained a similar aspect of the analytic relationship not yet in play. Furthermore, it seems that it was potentially helpful for Christina and me to be free to engage in a period of smooth sailing in order to develop a relationship sturdy enough to weather the primitive and chaotic affects, memories, fantasies, self- and other experiences and body states ensuing when previously dissociated relational constellations enter the analytic relationship. It also seems likely that when I changed cases in supervision, the container for the relational paradigm of abuse and frozenness was removed, subjecting the analytic dyad to these formerly unavailable self- and object experiences. Had my supervisor and I been engaged in exploring possible symmetrical and asymmetrical parallel processes in our work together, I might have been more prepared to recognize, hold, and process the transference–countertransference matrix of abuse and frozenness when it entered the analytic situation.

In the asymmetrical parallel process described in this vignette, the more chaotic, problematic, or primitive transference and countertransference constellation was enacted in the supervision and quite dissimilar to the relational paradigm found in the treatment. It could happen the other way around as well. For example, if supervisor and supervisee enjoy a particularly nurturing, warm, mutually fulfilling relationship while the supervisee and patient struggle with difficult or disruptive transference and countertransference responses, the possibility of an asymmetrical parallel process could be explored. Here, the supervisor and supervisee may be enacting a loving relational configuration currently dissociated from the treatment.

This relational model of parallel process proposes that parallel process is a two-way street in which relational patterns from either dyad can influence the other. A number of vignettes discussed here illustrate that point. We close this chapter with an unusual perspective on the reciprocal nature of parallel process, one offered by a patient. This example also depicts the kind of transferences patients develop toward their analysts' supervisors. When one of us (Frawley-O'Dea, 1997c) was a postdoctoral candidate, analytic work with Karen was presented to two very different supervisors. Karen, my (Frawley-O'Dea's) control patient, knew I was a postdoctoral student and also was aware that the tape recordings of our sessions were discussed in supervision. At the end of the second supervision, I stopped taping because I planned to introduce a new patient for the next year's supervision. After the taping came to a halt, Karen asked if our work still was being supervised and, after eliciting some of her thoughts on the matter, I acknowledged that I was not, at that time, presenting our work. Her response was immediate and emphatic. "Good," she said, "because I have to tell you—even though I liked your first supervisor really a lot, I think this last one was a jerk, and I hated what he or she did to us!"

Startled, I asked Karen to share more about her experience of the two supervisions. She related that she was sure the first supervisor was "loose, spontaneous, quick, and funny." She suspected that he or she had urged me to be more spontaneous and loose. "And you *were*," Karen said, "and it felt so good and made it safer and easier to be with you and to talk to you and be looser and more spontaneous myself!" The second supervisor was felt by Karen to have been more conservative, cautious, and less willing to share countertransference experiences and personal data. "You were still you, but you seemed less present and more careful, which scared me," she said, "*and* it was absolutely the worst on Wednesday, so I figured you must have been with your supervisor on Tuesday." She was correct about the day.

Obviously, there were a multitude of relational threads to untangle in all this, including Karen's transferences to the supervisors, her feelings about being a "guinea pig," elements of her transference to me that she projected outside the analytic dyad onto the supervisors, her unwillingness to bring any of this up until I was no longer in supervision, and more. Still, she also clearly experienced in parallel my own experiences of the two supervisions, albeit with significant exaggeration. In fact, however, I *also* felt safer and easier in the first supervisory relationship that did, indeed, emphasize spontaneity and use of the analyst's self in the treatment relationship (e.g., engaging in countertransference disclosure and even revealing certain personal information). In the second more difficult and conservative supervision, I felt less secure and more constrained. Interestingly, in neither supervision was much time spent on articulating the relationship developing between myself and my supervisor.

Karen's comments certainly suggest that both positive and negative relational constellations can transfer, or parallel, from supervision into the supervised treatment. Furthermore, this vignette highlights the potential worth of exploring a patient's transferences to the supervisor when the patient knows the analytic work is being supervised, or when the analyst and/or supervisor hears derivatives that the patient is aware of a third participant in the treatment.

Parallel process has been a richly debated psychoanalytic concept for many years. The model of parallel process described in this chapter strives to demystify the phenomenon and offers it as one potential thread to explore in unraveling the complex transference–countertransference configurations arising in and mutually influencing the supervisory and treatment dyads. The supervisor and supervisor who converse about their own relationship can ask themselves and each other the following questions: (1) What is the relational pattern currently in play in the supervisory relationship?; (2) what does it tell us about the relationship between this supervisee and this supervisor and their work together?; and (3) what, if anything, does it suggest to us about the transference and countertransference of the supervised treatment? A relational model of parallel process helps the supervisory dyad explore the third question in a systematic way.

CHAPTER 9

Contemporary Case Conference

As we noted in Chapter 2, psychoanalytic "supervision" had its origins in 1902, at the Wednesday night meetings of Freud and his followers. According to Gay's (1988) account, these free-wheeling meetings, which included case presentations, started off with high spirits and enthusiasm. However, some in the group grew weary of Freud's refusal to consider others' ideas. In addition, Gay observes, "The provocative subject matter of psychoanalytic inquiry, rudely touching on the most heavily guarded spots in the human psyche, was taking its toll and generating a pervasive irritability" (p. 177). Eventually, several members of the group grew discontent and left. Many modern-day case conferences struggle with similar issues: a leader who expects his views to prevail, and members who become disillusioned and resentful; a group process that becomes conflictual as emotionally loaded clinical material is discussed; and the flight of members from the group. In part, of course, this is because these are universal issues in groups. But in part it may also reflect the legacy of the dynamics of that initial group led by Freud.

In this chapter we reevaluate that inheritance and rethink case conference by bringing to bear relational theory, and contemporary understandings about groups and how they function. We start with an example of a case conference that illustrates some of the problems and limitations our model tries to address.

DIDACTICALLY ORIENTED CASE CONFERENCE

Ken was presenting Arthur, a patient in his late 40s, to a continuing case conference. The leader was an analyst, skilled in an ego psychological approach, who had been conducting case conferences for many years. Mindful of engaging the group in the teaching and learning process, she asked members to give their comments in turn after a session had been presented in full. Then, she gave her own perspective on the material. Rather than address differences of point of view, she let each member's comments stand alone. She did not invite participants' affective responses or free associations, but only their inferences about the patient. The leader's point of view was well articulated and elucidated a number of aspects of the patient's mind in terms of drive theory. During the early weeks, there was a sense of order and cognitive clarity in the structure of the conference as she used the case as an opportunity to teach about intrapsychic structure, defensive processes, psychopathology, and technique.

Ken was an experienced psychoanalytic therapist. Arthur, a professional and a divorced father of a teenage daughter, suffered from a moderate depression. At the time of Ken's presentation, Arthur's daughter was living with her more seriously depressed and self-destructive mother. Arthur felt that the situation was destructive for her and urged her to move in with him instead. The daughter refused to consider it, feeling enraged at her father for abandoning her mother, and not wanting her mother to feel abandoned a second time. Arthur became distraught about this, calling his daughter daily, urging her to free herself from her caretaking role with this difficult woman, but the daughter refused to accept his calls. Arthur felt defeated and hopeless.

The case conference leader expressed the view that Arthur had sacrificed his daughter to replace himself as caretaker of the mother/ex-wife, and that the therapist should confront him with his irresponsibility. She discussed the issue in diagnostic and technical terms, explaining why she felt the treatment could not be fully effective without such a confrontation. She thought that Arthur's narcissistic character pathology, which she felt his abandonment of his daughter represented, made him difficult to treat analytically.

Ken saw things differently. Not primarily struck with Arthur's narcissism, Ken instead identified with the anguish created by the impossible bind in which Arthur found himself. He felt Arthur's choices had been either to stay trapped in a destructive marriage or to find himself in his current dilemma with his daughter. Ken was impressed by the excruciating pain that Arthur's inability to help his daughter was causing him. He felt that confronting Arthur with his irresponsibility would only reinforce his tendency toward self-punitive guilt and self-reproach.

Thus, the case conference leader and the analyst were in clear disagreement. Such disagreements were not a subject of interest, however, to this case conference leader. She communicated implicitly that although different analytic therapists might see things differently, she did not feel it would be useful to take up the question of what the disagreements might mean. She calmly offered her perspective to the presenter and to the conference, and then left the members to do with it as they chose. However, tension developed in response to this important area of disagreement between the leader and the presenter, although it temporarily subsided after a few weeks, as the conference went on to other matters.

The issue later resurfaced, however. Despite Ken's strong initial disagreement with the leader's formulation, her point of view made an impact upon him, and he began to worry that he was being "too soft" on his patient, and that this would limit the possibilities of what might be accomplished in the treatment. This led Ken to confront Arthur in the terms that the leader had suggested, and he did so somewhat impulsively. As he reported the session to the group, it became apparent that the session had not gone well. The intervention seemed to precipitate a momentary rupture in their relationship. There appeared to be much that might be fruitfully explored about how and why things had unfolded in this way.

This case conference leader, however, responded again by refocusing on the patient, observing that the confrontation had not gone well because of the patient's character pathology. She raised no other questions about this clinical sequence and the group's participation in it, nor did she pick up on such issues when raised by group members.

This case conference leader's theory did not allow her to appreciate that her formulation might express her personal subjectivity and therefore resonate with only one aspect of the patient. She did not view her formulation as an imbedded response, saturated with aspects of transference–countertransference, and she did not realize that she might hold only one aspect of the truth rather than the whole truth. Her convictions about what was "true" about the patient naturally carried disproportionate weight in the minds of the presenter and other group members. Ken abandoned his own perspective on his patient and adopted the leader's, causing a disruption of his relationship with Arthur. The leader's theory provided no framework for stepping back and considering the variety of formulations offered by other members of the group and the presenter, and engaging in exploration that might have led to a more integrative and less disruptive understanding of the patient, the therapeutic relationship, and the conference process.

A relational perspective offers a framework for making sense of such events in both the case conference process and the therapeutic process. From this point of view, the leader and Ken could be understood to have identified with different aspects of Arthur's internal object world: the leader, with a self-critical aspect of Arthur, and Ken, with a part of Arthur that felt quite helpless and victimized. Ken's shift to confrontation thus represented his movement from one identification to the other. For Ken to speak from either position represented an enactment that would, ideally, eventually be processed in the therapy. From a relational perspective, the role of the case conference leader would be to help the presenter and the group to reflect on *both* views of the patient and to think about how both were true. Such efforts might have lead Ken to a fuller understanding of Arthur's complex and divided internal experience. It also would have allowed Ken to interpret both aspects of that experience to Arthur, which might have been easier for Arthur to make use of than Ken's sudden shift from one stance to another.

When group members' views are not welcomed into the formal conference setting, they often are expressed instead by subgroups outside of the conference. This did in fact occur in this conference. Although such extragroup conversations can provide some relief of unprocessed tensions, members may experience their outside-of-group insights into the group process as something that is split off from "real" analytic work and, consequently, be hampered in their efforts to integrate their countertransference experiencing analytically.

Members of this conference learned something intellectual about the patient and about technique. However, they missed an opportunity to learn experientially about all that might have emerged from the process of holding, valuing, and negotiating differences in the meanings that the leader, the presenter, and the various members attributed to the material, and about how to use it all in the service of creating an interpretation that will help the patient. It is our hope that our model of case conference, grounded in the principles of relational theory, and drawing upon the group process as a source of important information about the presented treatment's relational themes, can provide a fuller opportunity for learning.

PROCESS-ORIENTED (RELATIONAL) CASE CONFERENCE

A relational case conference is an analytic experience, not just a didactic one. It is a means of facilitating the learning of a craft rather than merely a means of communicating a body of knowledge. Just as the supervisory relationship is central to teaching and learning in individual supervision, the group process is central to teaching and learning in case conference. We therefore introduce our model by presenting some ideas from psychoanalytic group theory that we find useful in case conference.

Case Conference as a Group

The group supervisory situation differs from the dyadic situation in several ways that hold great potential for learning. In individual supervision, for example, it is easy for the supervisor to overlook his own impact upon the unfolding of the supervisory relationship, and because of the power differential between supervisor and supervisee, the supervisee may feel unable to point out this omission. However, in a group, a third party is always present to witness the interaction of any dyad. This presence of an observing third is a source of enormous potential for understanding the complex relational themes that unfold in any supervisory situation, if the leader's orientation gives members permission to notice and to comment. Thus, for example, when the case conference leader views the difficulties that the presenter is having with the patient as due to the patient's problems only, or to the presenter's problems only, or if the leader has a negative interpersonal impact on the presenter of which he is unaware, the rest of the group is there to observe and discuss the transaction.

The group supervisory situation also provides the possibility for a freer-flowing associative process than does the dyadic situation. In case conference, a kind of group brainstorming can take place that is richer and more emotionally immediate than what generally occurs in dyadic supervision. Just as two heads are often better than one, so multiple heads can be better still, if their emotional and cognitive synergies can be effectively channeled.

And finally, the group situation provides a marvelous opportunity for experiencing firsthand the reality that truth is perspectival, that there is no such thing as a single "objective" observer or a single valid narrative. Because case conference members inevitably have a variety of different responses to the same clinical material, individual conference members can learn to relinquish their search for an absolute "truth," and instead learn something about their own ways of organizing the world, and their own areas of sensitivity and insensitivity. They may also have an opportunity to observe and appreciate the process of negotiation, through which the group struggles to construct a single more or less coherent narrative from its members' multiple perspectives.

Using the Group Process on Behalf of Teaching and Learning

The idea that attending to group process in a case conference can facilitate and enrich the learning in that conference is certainly not new. Perhaps the first example of a case conference that explicitly made use of a group as something more than an efficient medium for didactic teaching came from Ferenczi's analysand, Balint. Balint (1957) ran a case conference for medical practitioners which Cooper and Gustafson (1985) describe as "not an expedient use of [supervisory] groups to address more individuals at once, not psychotherapy in disguise, but teaching about healing in a healing environment" (p. 15).

No case conference leaders are more familiar with group theory or understand better how to use the case conference process for teaching than those who specialize in group therapy. Group therapy supervisors value case conference as a method for supervising group therapy because it makes use of the isomorphisms between the clinical intervention to be taught (group therapy) and the teaching medium (case conference) (Altfeld and Bernard, 1997; Cooper and Gustafson, 1985). The process in the supervision group is assumed to parallel the process that is occurring in the therapy group (Altfeld and Bernard, 1997; Hilpert, 1995; Pfeffer, Epstein, and Herrara, 1989; Steadman and Harper, 1995). The regression-inducing, free-associative ambience of the supervision group facilitates the presenter's introduction into the conference process of her unconscious identification with those aspects of the patient(s) that she is having difficulty in consciously formulating. The supervision group is viewed as providing an opportunity to address and master those aspects experientially as well as cognitively.

Altfeld and Bernard (1997) give an example of a case conference for group therapists that was intended to maximize the regressive, affective, and experiential qualities of case conference, while minimizing its usual intellectual aspects. Their example defines the extreme case for how one may use case conference group process as the centerpiece of the teaching and learning experience. Here, the case conference leader systematically interrupted members who tried to offer formulations and asked instead for their feeling reactions to the material. The productive work done in this case conference resulted from the leader's capacity to contain, to encourage the development of, and, finally, to name the anxieties that were transmitted from patient to presenting therapist to group. Altfeld and Bernard's model of case conference demonstrates the power and value of skillful use of group process. However, negotiation about what degree of affective intensity is mutually acceptable to members and leader, crucial to a relational model of case conference, is missing from their approach. The leader expects members to tolerate levels of anxiety that are at times so high that they may interfere with learning.

Using Group Theory to Understand Difficulties in the Case Conference Process

Psychoanalytic group theory can be enormously helpful in understanding difficulties that inevitably arise in the case conference process. These difficulties may be formulated in terms of oedipal transferences, as Billow and Mendelsohn (1987) illustrate:

> The presenter may suddenly be perceived unconsciously [by the group] as the favored child, the newly discovered father, etc. . . . The therapist has powerful emotional reactions to the group-as-supervisor, and to particular individual group members as well. Thus a triangle exists, with the therapist being mutually influenced by the patient on the one side, and the supervisory group on the other. Perhaps, like the oedipal child, the presenter derives both excitement and frustration from the role of being the unexcluded middle. (p. 40)

The leader's sensitivity to the existence of such transferences, and ability to work with them, improves the process of a group that may otherwise become mired in anxiety and resistance, and unable to function effectively.

Kleinian theory, as developed by Bion, has added another dimension to understanding the irrational processes that interfere with pursuit of the group's task. Although case conference has a different task from the therapy groups for which Bion's theory was originally devised, or the self-study groups that were developed later (Bion, 1961; Rioch, 1970), the case conference leader can use ideas about *work groups* and *basic assumption groups* to address processes that get in the way of analytic understanding. Bion's (1961) ideas about groups are particularly relevant to our model because they are based in two-person psychology: In Bion's view, the leader is not an uninvolved observer of the group's problems but, rather, participates to some degree in their creation and maintenance.

For Bion (1961), the term "work group" describes a group in which members cooperate and put effort into accomplishing the group's task. For a case conference, the task might be defined as using the group process to increase analytic understanding of the patient and the treatment relationship. A work group is in good contact with reality and can tolerate frustrations and other painful affects evoked in the process of the work.

Bion (1961) contrasts work groups with three kinds *of basic assumption groups*, that is, three particular states of mind and modes of functioning into which groups fall that disrupt and oppose the cooperative reflectiveness of the work group. The three basic assumption groups that Bion describes are *dependency groups*, *fight–flight groups*, and *pairing groups*.

The *dependency* group operates on the unconscious assumption that there is someone, usually the group leader, upon whom all can depend to carry out the work that needs to be done. Although it is, of course, appropriate and realistic for case conference members to look to the leader as a source of special expertise, the case conference that is under the sway of this unconscious assumption of dependence becomes mired in an exaggerated form of childlike helplessness, losing track of its members' competence and ability to think independently. This group state of mind will often show itself in the tendency of the conference to look to the leader to advise the presenter about diagnosis and how to help the patient. There is little sense of mutuality in the interaction between leader and group members, and lively discussion of contrasting perspectives rarely occurs. Appreciation of the nature of dependency basic assumption groups can help to bring to life a case conference whose members have become passive and unable to think. Many case conference leaders allow themselves to be seduced into the role of "expert," feeling and behaving as if only they *did* in fact have the answers, and then blaming the group for its passivity. Understanding this dynamic allows the case conference leader to see a number of other possible options (Cooper and Gustafson, 1985). The leader's job is to become aware of his participation in the process, to refrain from colluding, and to invite the group to engage in self-reflection.

How one responds to a dependency basic assumption group, or to any basic assumption group, depends on many variables, of course, including the level of sophistication and the amount of anxiety in the group at the time. In order to keep anxiety at a level consistent with learning, an unsophisticated and anxious group requires more active participation from the leader and more tolerance for genuine dependence than does a more sophisticated and secure group. But knowing to ask the question, "How appropriate is it to go along with the dependent behavior of the group at this moment, or should this behavior rather become an issue that we inquire into together?" puts the case conference leader in a very different relationship to his group.

The *fight–flight* group operates on the unconscious assumption that an enemy exists inside or outside the group from whom it is necessary to defend itself or else flee. Persecutory anxiety and hostility are the dominant affects experienced by members—and leaders—under the sway of this basic assumption, and identifying the enemy and attacking it, or withdrawing from it, will appear to be a necessary means of maintaining security and managing anxiety. In a case conference, it is sometimes the presenter who comes to be identified as the enemy and is subtly or not-so-subtly attacked, although, on occasion, the group will cast the leader in the enemy role. Some case conferences that are gripped by a fight–flight dynamic appear superficially to be congenial but manage to seem so only by projecting the "enemy" outside of the group, and into the patient. The group—and leader—may then collude in an agreement to "blame the patient," unifying around a perception of the patient as difficult and untreatable. This strategy reduces tension in the case conference but defensively limits the group's ability to empathize with the patient and to reflect on other reasons for the therapeutic impasse. This seemed to be the case, for example, in the vignette of Arthur and Ken described earlier. The case conference leader may choose to bring the dynamic to the attention of the group and thus protect the group from actual flight, from psychological withdrawal, from attacking, or from becoming stuck in a defensive impasse.

The *pairing group*, the third basic assumption group, operates on the unconscious assumption that a couple within the group can bring forth a messianic child or idea that will save the group from its feelings of hate or despair. When in the grip of such an unconscious assumption, a group will often nominate one member to pair with the leader, or two group members to pair with each other, out of this unconscious hope. In case conference, one may notice a willingness to allow one group member to be specially engaged with the leader—talking with him, sitting next to him, and so on—without competitive challenge, and with an underlying sense of positive expectation. The leader can easily play into this dynamic, experiencing the nominated group member as special, and an erotic dimension can emerge in the pair, unconsciously encouraged by the rest of the group. This basic assumption tends to inhibit participants from taking responsibility for and addressing their difficulties directly, instead delegating responsibility for resolving them to the nominated pair and the messianic future. Also, a group member nominated by the group to pair with the leader may experience anxiety as a result of the role and accompanying erotic feelings that the group unconsciously encourages in her. This may lead to maladaptive defenses that interfere with learning, as was the case in a situation described in a paper by one of us (J. Sarnat, 1997). The leader's ability to reflect on his participation in the dynamic, and to bring the dynamic to the group's attention, can free the nominated member and the rest of the group to return to their task.

Bion's list of three basic assumption groups is not necessarily exhaustive. Another irrational process in which case conferences often engage might be called the *competitive group*. In such a group, members operate on the basis of the unconscious assumption that there is a prize to be won, in the form of the leader's praise and attention, and that only one member may win it. Groups in the grip of this basic assumption will have difficulty listening to one another and responding to and building upon one another's ideas. Creative brainstorming and group associative freedom will be stymied by members' needs to devalue or attack other contributions. In this mode, participants will also lose empathy for others' narcissistic vulnerabilities and learning needs, and feel pressured to show off what they know at the expense of other members. As with all basic assumption groups, the leader's ability to identify the dynamic, consider his collusion with it, and, if appropriate, bring it to the group's attention, can significantly shift the atmosphere in the conference.

Basic assumption groups are seen by Bionians as a form of group resistance, opposing growth, development, and particularly insight (Grinberg, Sor, and de Bianchedi, 1977). But in case conference, these irrational processes may also be viewed as meaningful enactments stemming from the presented case. Just as projective identification may be viewed as both a defensive effort to split off and disown an unwanted part of the self and an unconscious effort to communicate to the other a state that cannot be communicated through words, basic assumption life may be viewed not only as resistance but also as an important source of information for analytic processing. It is, of course, true that in case conference, as in all educational situations, we strive to encourage thinking, understanding, and making meaning rather than only the unconscious enacting of primitive states. But accepting the inevitability of the regressive experience of basic assumption life in case conference and its multiple sources in the intragroup and patient–presenter–group interaction can lead to a depth of learning that is not otherwise possible. Our model thus assumes that case conferences will strive to be "work groups" but also acknowledges that for significant periods of time, and for a number of different reasons, they will inevitably become "basic assumption groups" and that the alternation between these modalities can create a powerful opportunity for learning.

We now more fully describe and illustrate our process-oriented (relational) model of case conference.

The Model Described and Illustrated

Our model of case conference emphasizes the importance of creating a potential space that invites affectively engaged participation from supervisee, supervisor, and, eventually, patient, in which more becomes imaginable, sayable, and "playable" for all participants. By exploring the case conference group process, much can be learned about the therapeutic process. To the degree that it is safe to "know" ones feelings within the interpersonal field of the case conference, the presenter will also feel freed to "know" what is happening in the therapeutic relationship and to facilitate the patient's freedom to "know." A relational case conference leader works to create a learning environment in which affects and other experiences evoked by the patient, the presenter, or any aspect of the process, can be owned and acknowledged by members, without criticism or accusations of being "unprofessional."

The leader thus takes responsibility for nurturing a generative atmosphere within the conference. Yet he simultaneously recognizes the limits of what he alone can do. The leader views himself as involved in *co-creating* that atmosphere along with group participants. He also views himself as dependent upon the authorization of the case conference members themselves for much of the power that he does possess.

The leader makes no claim to knowing an ultimate "truth." Clinical truth is viewed as mutually negotiated and never finally settled. Sometimes, of course, the leader will function as "clinical expert," giving his personal view of the patient, the therapist's technique, and how the therapeutic process is unfolding. And depending upon the composition of the group, he will do so from a position of somewhat greater experience and expertise than other conference members. But his participation in the role of "clinical expert" is always tempered by his understanding that his view of what is happening in the case and in the conference is relationally imbedded, perspectival, and continually subject to revision. Thus, his contribution will become part of a developing series of understandings within the group rather than being a kind of "last word."

The relational case conference leader functions in a variety of roles. First, as a discussion leader, he encourages members to associate to the material and to express their ideas, then clarifies and synthesizes what the group comes up with, inviting the conference members to join him in this process. He also helps the group to remain open to possibilities and alternative hypotheses rather than allowing it to reach premature closure. He champions the case conference as a space for the interplay of ideas.

The case conference leader also makes a special effort to create a safe environment for the presenter. At times, this may mean that the leader uses his authority to set limits on a member's participation, if it threatens to impinge on the presenter's or other group members' sense of safety, or the group's potential space. He holds for the group the reality that the presenter has special knowledge of the patient, and thus special authority in this regard. At the same time, the case conference leader respects the perspectives of group members, who, by virtue of their more distant relationship to the patient, are free to have different experiences and to see different things. He does, however, insist that such dissenting views be respectfully and nondogmatically expressed. The case conference leader encourages participants to articulate what the treatment relationship *is* rather than to prescribe what it *should be*. When participants are tempted to tell the presenter what he should have done differently, the leader reminds the group that its primary job is to understand rather than to advise. Thus, he encourages members to maintain a playful and tentative relationship to their own reactions to the patient and the treatment, and to view these as being as much an expression of their own relational themes as they are instructive to the presenter. This stance of the leader helps to protect the potential space of the conference, as well as protecting the presenter from feeling overwhelmed, intruded upon, or wounded by members' comments.

In addition, the case conference leader plays the role of affective container, emotionally holding the group, and trying to put into words the strains that the group may feel pulled to act out in ways that threaten its ability to work. He not only addresses tensions between members and encourages the group to reflect upon them as more data to be understood, but also helps the group to consider its process in terms of basic assumption life, when this perspective seems likely to facilitate the work.

The leader also helps the group to think about its process in relation to the case. The data utilized in a relational case conference will be drawn not only from the presenter's process notes but also from the experience of all participants. He assumes that much of the important data will not be symbolically communicated by the presenter, but will show up instead in the affective states, associations, and enactments of any and all participants. He considers events in the group as a potential source of information about dissociated and unformulated aspects of the presented case, and using the concept of parallel process, works to make links between the experiences of members and the presented treatment.

The group process is viewed as the intersection of multiple

subjectivities, including those of the patient, the presenter, the members of the group, the leader, and possibly others. The group process is a composite of relational themes emerging between case conference members (including the leader), relational themes originating in the supervised treatment, and possibly themes from the presenter's analysis and the organization(s) in which the treatment and/or case conference are imbedded. These various themes exist in dialectal tension with one another, alternatively becoming foreground and background. Because there are multiple subjectivities in the room, each mind attuned to particular aspects of the case, a rich pastiche of affects, images, dissociative phenomena, and regressive experiences emerge within case conference, and the gathering up and exploring of these phenomena can deepen the presenter's understanding of her patient, herself, their interaction, and the broader contexts in which the treatment is imbedded.

Case conference is similar to a therapy group in that it is an analytic experience of depth, but differs in its task. Where a therapy group attempts to help patients to grow and develop in a global way, the case conference pursues two more specific goals. First, the case conference strives to facilitate the professional development of participants—their ability to generate and evaluate inferences about the patient and the treatment, their capacity to tolerate and to process analytically their own responses, and their development of analytic identities. Second, the case conference strives to help the therapist to help the patient.

A relational case conference, rather than being tightly structured, will instead allow for a free-flowing group process that facilitates the emergence of unconscious and affectively alive contents. Relatively unconstrained and unselfconscious material-generating periods will tend to alternate with more reflective material-processing periods. Negotiation of how the group will work is also an integral aspect of this free-flowing discussion process. Group members will be actively encouraged to speak up if the process begins to feel unsafe or if they begin to experience undue levels of anxiety. And the leader will actively monitor the presenter's comfort with the group's discussion, and will stand up for her if the group begins to become judgmental or critical.

The leader brings to the group's attention any rigid patterns that seem to hold the group back, such as directing all input to the presenter, as if she should accept and utilize all that is said; or directing all input to the leader, as if he were an expert whose approval is the primary aim; or only offering observations about the patient or therapist rather than also expressing one's own feelings. Such rigidities are sometimes an indication that unconscious anxieties and basic assumptions are dominating the process of the group.

Excerpts from two case conferences illustrate concretely this approach. The first vignette illustrates how a skillful relational case conference leader can make valuable use of potentially disruptive affective experiences that emerge within the group.

For 4 weeks, Mary presented Lisa, an intelligent, seriously disturbed woman in her 30s, to a case conference. Mary began her presentation by reading a summary of Lisa's life situation and problems. The conference learned from Mary that Lisa was given to hurting herself in multiple ways, leading on one occasion to a medical crisis. Mary presented in a matter-of-fact way a long list of Lisa's mutilation strategies. She read this material, rather than speaking extemporaneously to the group, as she had been invited to do.

When the group fell silent in response to this recital, the conference leader inquired about its reactions. Some members of the group expressed disgust, revulsion, terror, fatigue, and difficulty thinking. Others expressed interest in the challenges of the case and fascination with Lisa's bizarre symptoms.

Toward the end of the first meeting, Mary presented a recent session. The conference members wondered whether Mary was in tune with Lisa's feelings and therapeutic needs. In particular, a question was raised about Mary's decision to extend the session at the last minute, at Lisa's request. The group felt that Mary should have provided a firm time boundary, particularly given Lisa's tendency to act out her impulses. It seemed hard for the group to "get" the reasons why Mary behaved as she did in the session. The leader, however, encouraged the group to try to understand why things might be unfolding as they were, rather than recommending how things should go differently. He also focused the group on verbalizing and trying to understand their own reactions to the material.

In the second conference meeting, the leader invited the conference members to begin with reflections on the experience of the previous week. Members' associations focused on the meaning of Mary's style of presentation. One member suggested that perhaps Mary had been vicariously traumatized by this patient's material, which might account for the relatively affectless way that she presented it to the

group, including her choice to read the list of self-mutilation strategies. Others took it a step further and wondered if she might also have
been identifying with the perpetrator/aggressor within the patient, trying, unconsciously, to get the group to experience some of the distress
that she herself had been unable to let herself feel in listening to Lisa's
accounts.

Mary then told the group she realized that presenting so much
traumatic material might have been hard for members to tolerate.
She said that she herself was unaware of much feeling about the material, since Lisa presented herself in session in such an unthreat-
ening way. The group reflected on how much freer participants in
the conference might feel to experience the full impact of Lisa's self-
destructive behavior, and the aggression that Lisa had split off, than
was Mary, who was isolated in an ongoing, face-to-face relationship
with Lisa.

When Mary presented two new hours in this second meeting, the
group had a very different reaction to them. The group felt that Mary
was more in tune with what her patient needed and could tolerate
from her, feeling that Mary was enacting the role of mother superior/
confessor, and that this devoutly Christian patient was responding
favorably to this, while a more typical analytic stance would almost
certainly have led her to flee treatment.

When the group members tried to make sense of this surprising
shift in their perception of the therapeutic dyad, two related hypotheses were proposed. First, they wondered if Mary's ability to respond to
her patient may have increased once she had begun to utilize the conference as a container for her unmetabolized countertransference responses to her patient. Group members could "store" these responses
until it became possible for the therapist to use them within the treatment. In addition, the group members wondered if their own ability to
empathize with Mary's work might have increased after they had processed the distress and defensiveness that the traumatic material had
aroused in them in the initial meeting.

A variety of intensely disturbing affects were experienced by
members of this conference. Critical, judgmental reactions occurred
alongside emotional withdrawal, a kind of fight–flight dynamic in
response to the anxiety that this presenter and her patient evoked in
the group. The group's response might also be viewed as the enactment of a defense against a dissociated sadomasochistic transference–

countertransference. The presenter could not verbalize her counter-transference reactions, and instead unconsciously induced her unsymbolized affects into the group. The group leader provided a strong holding presence and, rather than colluding with this dynamic, was able to maintain a steady analytic attitude toward the case, the presenter, and the group. He persisted in trying to understand "what was" rather than joining with the pull of the group to tell the presenter "what should be."

The presenter was able to make use of the group as a container for troubling experiences that had been unthinkable and unspeakable, and then, as a result, to function more effectively with her patient. If conference members had been confined to trying to understand the patient and the therapeutic process, focusing, for example, exclusively on the presenter's process notes, without attending to their own experience, they would most likely have come to impasse or, worse, become hurtful to presenter and patient.

We close with an extended excerpt from an 8-week case conference, observed primarily from the point of view of one participant. This vignette shows how themes from the presented treatment parallel into the case conference. There, they are initially enacted by the group, then eventually processed, thus providing the presenter with help in mastering and symbolizing a previously unarticulated counter-transference response.

In the second meeting of the conference, Carl began to present his work with Sara, a woman in her late 20s whose stepfather had abused her throughout her childhood. Her mother had had recurrent severe illnesses that required hospitalization. Sara was the child who cared for mother and held the household together. Despite periods of substance abuse, Sara had done well in school and had established a successful career in real estate. She was clearly a "survivor." She came to treatment because of her inability to sustain an intimate relationship and her wish to marry and have a child. Carl had been seeing Sara in intensive psychotherapy for several months.

Carl presented detailed process from two sessions. In the first, there seemed to be a light and playful mood in their interaction, although the material was rather superficial. In the next, Sara revealed her sexual feelings and fantasies toward Carl, who actively interpreted those feelings and related them to Sara's childhood experience of abuse.

Janice, a member of the conference, reacted to the second session by becoming anxious, and angry with Carl. She felt that he was out of touch with how sensitive and exposing the material that Sara brought up in the second session would be for an adult survivor of childhood sexual abuse, and she felt protective and worried for Sara. Janice felt reluctant, however, to express these feelings in the case conference because they were critical and would likely be experienced by Carl as an attack. She realized that she might be caught up in some kind of group process, but she had no sense of how to get out of it. The best that she could do was to wait to see if others might perhaps raise the issue with more grace than she felt capable of herself. However, perhaps not surprisingly, no one in the group seemed to feel any freer to speak than she did, and her concerns were not addressed.

As the conference meeting proceeded, Janice felt increasingly frustrated. She kept struggling to figure out what was going on in the conference and how it related to the hour with the patient, but she could not think clearly about it. She found herself wondering about the purpose of the conference: Whose needs was it intended to meet? Carl's? Sara's? Her own and those of other group members? She kept hoping that the leader would intervene and comment on the process as well as the case material. Janice began to feel, although she could not put it into words until later, that there was no protective mother in either the hour with the patient or in the conference. She finally decided to speak up, hoping to engage the group and the leader in "helping" Carl to become more sensitive to Sara.

Janice told Carl about her concerns and how she thought he ought to work with Sara; she spoke not so much from her own experience, but in a "supervisory" fashion. He responded, not surprisingly, by becoming quiet and wary. Tension developed in the group. A basic assumption group appeared to be developing. Fight–flight dynamics, as well as the reverberations of trauma, were interfering with the capacity of the group members to work together.

At this point, the leader tried to address some of the anxieties that dominated the group. She asked Carl about his reaction to the group's comments, and when he expressed concern about being judged for the way he had worked with Sara, she assured him that her interest was in understanding whatever interaction had developed between them, not in judging it as right or wrong. She took the position that the analytic dyad's particular idiom had evolved for important reasons that it might be useful to articulate. He and the group seemed to relax somewhat, but Janice continued to feel agitated and guilty about the impact of her comments on Carl as the meeting ended. Interestingly, as she and Carl were getting into their cars, outside of the "basic assumption group atmosphere," Janice was able to speak to Carl more directly about her feelings of agitation and frustration, and to acknowledge to Carl that her comments had been hurtful to him. He responded to her with interest and a suggestion that they discuss further what had happened when the case conference met again.

In the next meeting, the leader started by inviting members to discuss their reactions to the previous meeting. Carl and Janice were then able to bring the essence of their postgroup conversation into the case conference. It became clear that other members had had a variety of different responses to what had transpired, but that the experiences of confusion, chaos, and cautiousness to avoid hurt and anger were generally shared. These experiences were articulated and clarified by the leader. The group moved toward more open and direct expressiveness, with one member speaking, for example, of how her experience in the group brought to mind experiences with her own psychotic mother. Carl let the group know that these direct expressions of countertransference feelings were much more useful to him than advice about working with the patient.

Once the loss of a work group atmosphere was processed by group members, and a work group atmosphere began to reemerge, it became possible for them to articulate some of the relational themes of the treatment that seemed to have been played out the previous week in the case conference process. In particular, the paralleling of the absent mother–motherless child and abuser–abused relational themes into the case conference process was noted. Coming back to the material with increased distance, and with the help of the leader's intervention, group members were able to think about and make use of what had been enacted. Identifying the here-and-now experience of this abuser–abused paradigm in the group (i.e., Janice's inability in that moment to find a "nonabusive" way to speak to Carl) helped Carl to see how the same paradigm might be operating in his relationship with Sara. What Janice and the rest of the group could not find a useful way to *tell* him, but could only reenact, the group members could now understand and articulate in a way that was useful to Carl.

What was crucial in this discussion was the leader's ability to shift the focus of the conference from discussing the case itself to discussing the process in the group. Her openness to honest expression of feeling, and her nondefensiveness in receiving feelings related to herself (including Janice's feeling of being neglected/abandoned by her) set an example for other members of the group. Her ability to do this without criticism or judgment created a space in which group members could work together to understand the group's dynamics and how these reflected and illuminated otherwise inaccessible aspects of the case, including important unconscious transference–countertransference paradigms. A framework had been established for processing future difficulties. But the issue was not resolved in any final way during this second meeting. Members of the group continued to experience conflict in owning and expressing their negative reactions to the clinical material, and, thus, they continued to have difficulty communicating with Carl.

In the eighth and final meeting, Carl started by expressing frustration with his relationship to Sara. As he had continued to present her to the group, he had become more aware that he rarely felt free to think during the hours, and rarely had the creative associations with her that he had with most patients. He was realizing, with the group's help, that she kept him off balance by sudden shifts in the hour, and by her frequent cancellations. He said that he was becoming increasingly aware of how difficult it was for him to talk to her about many things, including this frustration with their process.

Group members then discussed how their own sense of frustration might be understood—in part—as a parallel process. Throughout the weeks, although the leader and the group members had explicitly committed themselves to creating a space for free expression of thoughts and feelings, this had somehow often been impossible. Group members realized that despite their best conscious efforts, their comments continued, intermittently, to be expressed in judgmental terms, which made them difficult for Carl to use. They saw how, in reaction to Carl's apparent feelings of hurt and anger, they had become increasingly anxious and guilty, and even constrained, creating a vicious cycle. Yet even as this discussion unfolded, the sense of frustration and constriction persisted in the group.

Then, the leader made a final effort to communicate to Carl and the group her understanding of the transference–countertransference resistance that she felt dominated the field between Carl and Sara, a resistance that blocked their ability to communicate deeply with one another about important feelings. But Carl could not use this interpretive intervention either. The leader was distressed by Carl's seeming deflection of her intervention, but instead of backing off, as group members had repeatedly done, she persisted this time. "I know this is a part of my own countertransference, but it's also my real feeling and so I'm going to tell you anyway. THAT PISSES ME OFF!!!!" She said this with intensity but somehow also managed to communicate her ongoing connection to Carl. The atmosphere of the group then shifted. Renewed energy and a sense of freedom unexpectedly arrived. Both the group and Carl seemed to become more present, and he seemed to "get" what the leader and the group members had been unable to communicate clearly until then.

What had happened? From one perspective, the leader had succeeded in straddling a paradox that had stymied the group until that moment. She had understood that her frustrated feelings were part of a larger relational matrix, and she had also owned them and inhabited them as her personal experience. She had found a way to express strong feelings without being abusive or destructive and, in so doing, had freed the group—and Carl—to begin to do the same. Until that moment, all of the leader's and the group's efforts to connect the stuck process in the conference to the stuck feeling in the treatment had remained intellectual and made little difference in Carl's or the group members' experience. But the leader's freedom to own and express affect broke the spell and allowed the group to *experience* what had been impossible to teach didactically.

Group members then struggled to put into words what had happened. Both Carl's inhibition with his patient and the group's parallel inhibition with him in confronting a lack of contact had suddenly been put into bold relief by the leader's freedom to express herself affectively. Group members linked their inhibition to worries about aggression feeling abusive, which also led to deeper understanding of one of the sources of inhibition in the presented treatment.

The leader's participation in this session demonstrates something important about authority relations in a relational case conference. The leader's "outburst" was ultimately freeing rather than traumatic because of her clarity about her role as an imbedded participant rather than an authoritative and objective observer. She kept her own reactions in perspective, just as she kept participants' reactions in perspective: They were her own, she had a right to them, and she did not experience them as so powerful that they could traumatize. This was exactly the stance that group members had difficulty taking with Carl, that Carl was having difficulty taking with his patient, and that his patient had had difficulty taking throughout her life.

In this example, once again, the leader and the group members struggled to process in the group what could not be processed by the presenter in the therapy. This case conference experience was not an easy one, and the issues introduced from the treatment were challenging for this particular conference. However, a degree of understanding developed, along with increased emotional freedom, as countertransference blocks that had limited the therapist's ability to work were repeated within the process of the group, and partially articulated and worked through in the group.

Case conference can be one of the most difficult experiences in clinical training, fraught with the potential for the presenter and other group members to feel attacked and narcissistically injured. Given the tendency of group members to get carried away with their own affects and processes, case conferences can feel, at times, like a kind of powder keg waiting to go off. The choices that leaders make about structuring their conferences—such as whether to tightly structure the conference, and whether to encourage examination of group process—are often motivated by efforts to cope with anxiety about these powerful forces.

The case conference leader who works from a relational model is able to view these forces with less anxiety and more interest. Affective experiences, rather than being considered a distraction from the primary focus of the conference, are at the heart of the conference's work. The challenge to the case conference leader is to find a way to allow these experiences to be safely and constructively represented within the conference, to hold these experiences, and to help the group to work with them analytically, in order to better understand the patient, the therapist, and the therapeutic dyad's relationship. In the context of a well-contained group setting, associative freedom and the regressive potential of groups can present an opportunity for the expression of dissociated and otherwise unavailable aspects of the therapeutic dyad's experience, and an opportunity for transformation. The presenting therapist and the rest of the group can then see those affects and relational themes played out in front of them, and can learn both from watching and participating in the unfolding drama.

Conclusion

The Supervisory Dyad and Beyond

Psychoanalytic supervision and, indeed, any supervision, is about voices. It is about the supervisor's voice and the supervisee's voice and the patient's voice. Sometimes, these three voices move together in mutually influenced dialogue; sometimes one sounds in monologue, unsure of being heard or understood; sometimes they clash in a jarring dissonance of tone and pitch.

When a given supervision goes well, patient, supervisee, and supervisor find ways to co-narrate treatment and supervisory relationships that enable the patient to give voice *to* his life and to assume a voice *in* his life that is rich, full, and meaningful. When things go well, the patient's voice becomes more uniquely his own. Yet, at the same time, its accent and range reflect internalization of the therapist's voice and, in some indeterminate way, the supervisor's voice as well. Similarly, the supervisee develops a voice that is more uniquely her own, yet within which are detectable nuances, accents, and dialectical tones internalized through her clinical and supervisory encounters.

Ultimately, then, psychodynamic supervision is about therapists finding and refining their voices through the co-created conversations they have with their patients and supervisors. More broadly, clinical training in general, and psychoanalytic training in particular, is about analysts shaping their voices through the intersubjective experiences of their classes, personal analyses, supervisory encounters, collegial relationships, professional activities, and work with patients. All of these activities, however, are held within organizations—institutes, training program, colleges, and universities—that in turn are loosely linked through membership in and identification with the larger psychoanalytic community. The organization that sponsors any individual's training and supervision influences, often in inchoate ways, the freedom and flexibility with which patient, supervisee, and supervisor are able to put voice to a full range of thoughts, affects, body states, and fantasies relating to their work. If we take seriously the links between the supervisory dyad and the relational forces at play within the community in which the supervision takes place, we come to appreciate the profound impact of that more diffuse relational matrix on the voices of supervisor, supervisee, and patient. In this conclusion, we consider the interrelationship between the supervisory dyad and the organization that sponsors it. We also consider the mutual influence of supervisory dyads, organizations, and the wider psychoanalytic community.

Wherever supervision takes place, the sponsoring organization assumes a presence within the supervisory relationship. Pizer (1999), says it well: "Just as the supervisor represents a powerful third tacit presence in the consulting room with the candidate and the analysand, so does the internalized institution pose an important presence as a third point of reference for the supervisor who is never, in this sense, alone with a supervisee" (p. 8). Both members of the supervisory dyad inevitably respond both consciously and unconsciously to the ambience, anxieties, and preferred defenses of a particular organization. If the voices of the all supervisory participants are to grow strong and clear, it is up to the supervisor to attend to the organizational context in which she finds herself, to reflect with her supervisee upon its impact, and to consider that impact in refining her supervisory technique.

Taking the impact of the organizational context into account in one's own supervisory practice, however, is not enough. As members of individual organizations and of the wider professional community, supervisors also need to recognize and speak about those aspects of training organizations and of the broader culture of psychoanalysis that support training efforts and those aspects that detract (Kernberg, 2000). From the inception of psychoanalysis, psychoanalytic training has been conducted too often within a milieu characterized by power jockeying and competing claims by various schools of thought that they and only they carry the torch of psychoanalytic truth. As both Balint (1948) and Slavin (1997) emphasize, psychoanalytic training frequently has resembled more closely the initiation of clerics into religious dogma than the stimulation of questions, challenges, and creative new ideas. Slavin comments that this method of psychoanalytic training expresses "a search for an almost magical connection to the founders, virtually through a direct, generational laying on of hands" (p. 810). Slavin attributes the substantial limitations and rigidities that he observes among his psychoanalytic colleagues to such cultural pathology. These rigidities, intergenerationally transmitted through the training process, limit the creativity and flexibility of our field.

The best and most creative supervision takes place when the supervisor trusts her organizational structure to support her ability to use her voice uniquely and creatively, and to encourage her supervisees to do the same. It is especially important for the supervisor to feel that she can openly consult with peers and even more senior colleagues when she wants advice about a supervisory conflict or treatment issue that arises in the supervision about which she feels unsure. The supervisor very much needs to feel that her organizational community can tolerate variance amid and even deviance from the dominant tongue and tone spoken within that culture, while still maintaining appropriate professional standards and limits. For the supervisor to continue to grow and to refine her own voice as a clinician, supervisor, and community member, she must be able to rely on her organization to be a facilitating environment that is willing to and capable of holding a tension between conformity and deviation; between old and new; between the experimental and the tried and true. When the organization fails to hold, challenge, protect, and expect from the supervisor, that failure almost certainly is woven into the fabric of the supervision in a way that squelches the voices of patient, supervisee, and supervisor alike.

Equally important is an organization's capacity to express confidence in its supervisees and its therapists, and to tolerate the persecutory anxieties that inevitably are evoked in the course of this difficult work, without turning against the vulnerable student or her supervisor. When things go poorly, the restrictiveness of some psychoanalytic cultural norms, combined with anxieties active within the organization, can create a climate of paranoia and a clamping down on the freedom to speak with a unique and nonconformist voice. Two examples of organizations that struggled in different ways with these issues, and the impact that their struggles had upon supervisor and supervisee, follow.

Zoe was a psychologist in a Community Mental Health Center. She was a very recent graduate of a clinical psychology doctoral program and had been hired by the Center after completing her internship there with very positive evaluations. About 2 months into her permanent employment, a patient she had been seeing for 6 months, and about whom she had been talking in supervision, committed suicide. Zoe was devastated on many levels and, among many emotions and experiences of self and other, felt responsible for and ashamed about her patient's death.

From the day of her patient's suicide, the organization provided strong support for Zoe. Her supervisor spent most of that afternoon with her reviewing the case, allowing her to give voice to her feelings and fantasies, and supporting her clinical skills. He also made it clear to her that if anything had been "missed" in the treatment, he was in part responsible. Furthermore, he committed to Zoe that they would continue to revisit the clinical and supervisory work on this case until they felt that they understood as much as possible about the patient and her suicide.

That same afternoon, the Commissioner of Mental Health for the Center's geographic region, who was acquainted with Zoe's work, stopped by to offer his condolences and to express his continued confidence in Zoe's clinical skills. When she tearfully asked, "What if we get sued?" he responded, "I expect that we'll get sued. We always get sued no matter the circumstances. That's why we have insurance." The Commissioner also checked in on Zoe's supervisor to see how he was doing with Zoe and with his own feelings about the suicide. Later that day, and over the next several days, a number of staff members shared with Zoe and her supervisor stories of patients or loved ones who had killed themselves. These staff members provided great support and opportunities to talk for both Zoe and her supervisor.

Several weeks after the suicide, a psychological autopsy was held at the Community Mental Health Center. Zoe had provided a case write-up that her supervisor had helped her think through. Her supervisor attended the meeting at which most administrative and clinical officials of the county mental health system were present. It was made clear to Zoe that the purpose of the meeting was to review the case carefully to determine what, if anything, might have been done differently; to see if there was something to be learned from this case that might be applicable to other situations; and to help Zoe to begin to close the case officially and emotionally. The way the meeting was conducted left Zoe feeling that her healing was as important to the committee members as their clinical, ethical, and legal concerns.

At the end of the meeting, the committee concluded that Zoe's work with the patient had met professional standards. They felt that the suicide had been part of a long-term plan by the patient, one she had chosen not to share with anyone, and thus was not something that could have been prevented. The committee went out of its way to support both Zoe and her supervisor in their work with the patient and their presentation to the committee. At the same time, they instructed Zoe and her supervisor as to what was appropriate to say to whom about the patient, her death, and their own feelings. Thus, the committee also represented the interests of the Community Mental Health Center in a direct and straightforward way.

Several months later, Zoe was asked to join an interdisciplinary committee established to review cases with which individual clinicians, their supervisors, or treatment team leaders had questions or concerns. This committee gave therapists and supervisors an opportunity to consult with a wider group about especially challenging cases in an atmosphere of collegiality and free-ranging discussion. Its formation was one of the creative and constructive consequence of the tragedy of Zoe's patient's suicide.

Clearly, the organization in which Zoe's clinical work and supervisory relationship were conducted was one whose culture was infused with respect for, openness to, and compassion toward its members. From the Commissioner of Mental Health on down to junior staff, the intersubjective atmosphere was both holding and creatively challenging. Its members were viewed as capable and deserving of support. The organization stood ready to listen to the voices within it, to assist all voices in being heard, and, thus, to further the development and refinement of individual and subgroup voices contained within it. In order to do so, the organization was called on to contain and process enormous feelings of guilt, shame, and persecution rather than leaving them for the vulnerable new therapist and her supervisor to cope with alone.

Wheelis (1999), in a paper that provides an unusually candid glimpse of her trials as a nonconformist candidate in a traditional psychoanalytic institute, describes her training in an organization that was, in her experience, less able to provide the kind of holding Zoe's did. Because of difficulties tolerating multiple perspectives on what constitutes "analysis," as well as persecutory anxiety that dominated the organization at that moment, Wheelis described undergoing a variety of subtle attacks, innuendos, and undermining responses as she presented her first control case to supervisors and case conferences within her institute.

Wheelis's control case, although it did not involve a suicide, appeared to be equally problematic for this traditional institute because of the degree of disturbance that the patient evidenced, and the resulting need to work with the patient in a nontraditional analytic way. Indeed, the first supervisor that Wheelis approached declined to supervise the case, saying that the patient, Michael, was "too ill," and that the case was "too difficult," a response that Wheelis felt was a rejection of her and her clinical judgment. One can wonder whether anxieties stemming from this institute's narrow definition of what constitutes "true analysis," reverberating with pressures from the broader psychoanalytic community as to how one establishes one credentials as "a real analyst" or "real analytic supervisor," may have contributed to this supervisor's unwillingness. Would accepting the task of supervisor lead to colluding with both the candidate and the patient in doing something less than "true analysis"? Would the supervisor's judgment be questioned for agreeing to supervise such a control case?

However, despite this supervisor's assessment of Michael as "unanalyzable," and his apparent disapproval of Wheelis for choosing to offer analysis to this patient, he did give her the names of two other supervisors known for their willingness to work with "the so called widening scope patient" (p. 2). One of these supervisors agreed to supervise her analytic work with Michael, saying "with unmistakable passion and enthusiasm, 'By all means—it's his only hope' " (p. 3).

Successful engagement of a supervisor for her work with Michael, however, was not the end of Wheelis's difficulties. As she presented her work with Michael in case conferences, she was met with persistent criticism of both her selection of this patient for analysis and the way in which she worked with him. Several colleagues suggested that Wheelis was endangering her standing in the institute by working with this patient in some nontradtional analytic ways.

Despite the skepticism about and criticism of Michael's analysis, when Wheelis's work with the patient was actually reviewed by the institute's training committee, it was found to be satisfactory, and she was authorized to begin her next control case. However, during the postmeeting feedback session with the committee's chair, after receiving a number of thoughtful and constructive comments on her work, Wheelis

> was taken aback when she [the committee chair] commented that while she thought my work with Michael was good, she didn't think it was an analysis. She finished with a caution that I should be careful to protect my reputation. (p. 11).

In addition, when Wheelis later shared the paper cited here with her supervisor, he told her, "The other side to your story . . . is that I too have been criticized by other training analysts who feel I am not supervising an analysis" (p. 12).

In a postscript to her paper, Wheelis writes:

> Michael continues in analysis to this date. When I applied for certification there was some discussion about whether I should write up Michael as one of the required cases. . . . In the end I decided not to include him as one of my cases. My supervisor felt that I would just be asking for trouble. (p. 12)

How do a supervisor and a supervisee find their authentic voices in the context of such powerful organizational dynamics? The supervisor in this instance provided as much support, protection, and containment to his supervisee as any supervisor could, absorbing criticisms from his colleagues without passing them along to his supervisee and advocating her right to treat this difficult patient when other supervisors in the institute felt he was "unanalyzable." But he could not, ultimately, insulate Wheelis from the effects of the institute's anxieties and its narrow views of the analytic process. At one point, at a moment when Wheelis was struggling with acute distress about whether she would be allowed to progress within her institute, Michael accused her of pulling away from him, and she acknowledges in her paper that she felt he was absolutely right. Despite her efforts to the contrary, the organization's dynamics inevitably made an impact upon her relationship with her patient. Her vibrant voice had been dampened, and her patient knew it.

In this vignette, no one died: in fact, the patient improved greatly during his analysis. Yet, Wheelis's clinical work and supervision were impinged upon. Pizer (1999), commenting on Wheelis's paper, expresses his dismay at the organizational pressure under which this supervisory dyad had to labor. Interestingly, he uses the same language of religious initiation used by Balint (1948) and Slavin (1997) when he calls the implied judgments against Wheelis and her supervisor "whispers in the corridors of excommunication" (p. 11).

As a result of these organizational pressures, the kinds of open, heated but respectful discussions of real differences of opinion that characterize the most lively learning environments apparently could not take place in this institute at this time. How it might have stimulated true dialogue if Wheelis and her supervisor had jointly presented the clinical and supervisory material at an institute forum! What voices could have been heard! Such interchange can only happen, of course, when the ambience of an organization allows it to listen, to explore, to discuss, and to disagree within a context of collegial respect for and trust in each member of the organization. Meltzer (1992) puts it well:

> There are problems of organization and community where the borderland between friendly and hostile, communication and action, governing and ruling, opposing and sabotaging become obscure. . . . I would pose the problems involved as how to govern without ruling; how to communicate without acting; how to oppose without sabotaging; how to remain friendly when in disagreement. (pp. 153–154)

Without an atmosphere that is capable of holding and sustaining creative tensions at Meltzer's borderlands, organizational cultures can devolve into either compliance with a "company line" or a cacophony of voices, none listening to any other. In both cases, creativity is stifled, the possible is foreclosed, and meaning is attacked or destroyed.

We want to emphasize here that although organizations that find themselves, for whatever reason, in the grips of a rigid and judgmental dynamic do not facilitate the kind of supervisor/supervisee development that we value, neither does a facilitative organizational culture mean an endlessly indulgent one. In an open and flexible organizational system, there is room for sharp disagreements and passionate debate. There is also a need for limits that protect the overarching goals of the organization. If one joins an organization, institute, or training program, there is some responsibility to hold, to protect, and to facilitate the voice of the organization at the same time that one is held, protected, and facilitated. A maverick who is provocative or divergent just to be provocative or divergent speaks with no more authentic a voice than a compliant reciter of dogmatic litany. The organization ultimately can be only as respectful, tolerant, playful, and curious as the individuals who comprise it. It is the commitment of the individual to the organization, and of the organization to the individual, to negotiate mutually and to renegotiate continually expectations, limits, and possibilities that maximize the potential for creative interchange.

Analytic organizations, like supervision, are currently in transition. Despite the historical problems of power and defensiveness inherent in many psychoanalytic institutes and training programs, the same sociocultural and political trends that are converging on the supervisory relationship are also reaching into the organizations in which supervision takes place. For example, many institutes have recently expanded their definition of the analytically treatable patient to encompass populations most traditionalists would find inaccessible to psychodynamic approaches. These include sexual trauma survivors, substance abusers, the eating disordered, and inner-city, lower-socioeconomic-status patients whose lives are replete with real and serious challenges that coexist with their unique character structures and pathologies. At the same time, analytically oriented programs are becoming more open to other treatment modalities and are increasingly willing to incorporate them into their treatment and, thus, supervisory endeavors. These include referring patients for adjunctive psychopharmacological treatment, couple or family therapy, group therapy, or even integrating cognitive-behavioral techniques into a treatment when these can assist in expediting symptom relief. Furthermore, psychoanalytic training programs are stretching to serve a more geographically diverse constituency. Traditionally clustered on the East and West Coasts and in Chicago, new institutes have sprung up in Minnesota, Colorado, Texas, Oklahoma, and even on the Internet, where the didactic portion psychoanalytic training can be accessed on-line, with supervision often conducted by phone. These efforts to democratize psychoanalysis reflect postmodern shifts regarding decentralization of power and the value of multiple voices and perspectives.

Just as supervisory relationships bear the intersubjectively mediated influence of the organizational cultures in which the supervision takes place, individual psychoanalytic organizations and psychodynamically oriented training programs inevitably influence and are influenced by the wider psychoanalytic community represented by professional journals, books, conventions, meetings, and the various psychoanalytic Internet sites. Here, too, things are beginning to change.

For many years, one could pick up an issue of any psychoanalytic journal and be reasonably certain what authors would be featured, because those voices were the ones most usually heard in that publication. Similarly, meetings of professional associations, such as the American Psychoanalytic Association or the Division of Psychoanalysis (39) of the American Psychological Association, seemed year after year to showcase the same voices in lead roles and in supporting parts. The "old-boy network" was alive and well, and living in psychoanalysis as it was in many sectors of society, and, as in those other areas of sociocultural and political organization, the old-boy network often obstructed the new, the innovative, and the dissident. Recently, however, new names are appearing in existing journals, new journals have appeared, and new names and faces are on the speaker rosters of meetings and conventions, all suggesting that Balint's (1948) wish that all psychoanalytic languages be heard with respect is nearing fulfillment.

In the first issue of the new century, Altman and Davies (2000), recently appointed editors of *Psychoanalytic Dialogues: A Journal of Relational Perspectives*, write:

> The issues of diversity in psychoanalytic theory and technique and the relationship between psychoanalytic politics and the evolution of psychoanalytic ideas are complex. We believe that the health and vitality of psychoanalysis, of any discipline, is predicated on and not threatened by the vigor of respectful intellectual debate. . . . Of course, there is sometimes a fine line between fostering awareness of differences and contributing to divisiveness. Divisiveness, the highlighting of differences in the service of political ends, battles over turf, can be recognized by a lack of respect for the ideas of others, a failure to cite relevant work of people from other groups, an attitude of dismissiveness and contempt. . . . We are eager to publish articles

that rigorously challenge the relational perspective. We will also re-
double our efforts to seek new voices, to help new authors develop
"first papers," to leave space for the special kind of creativity that comes from those who are trying to "speak" for the first time. (pp. 2–3)

Jay Greenberg (personal communication, March 2000), editor of *Contemporary Psychoanalysis*, echoes Altman and Davies when he reports
that that journal's editorial board recently made an explicit decision to
publish more new voices in the journal and to help authors of first papers to get into press. In addition, Greenberg said his journal has been
receiving many more submissions from newer analysts and he attributes this to the loosening up of theoretical structure and the institu-
tional and social changes in psychoanalysis and in the wider society
over the past 10 to 15 years. Concomitant with the commitment of
existing journals to invite and encourage new voices in their pages,
new journals have appeared that speak to the broadening of what is
welcome under the umbrella of psychoanalysis, for example, *Gender
and Psychoanalysis*, *Studies in Gender and Sexuality*, the *Journal of Neuro-
Psychoanalysis*, and the *Journal of Studies in Applied Psychoanalysis*.

As psychoanalysis enters its second century, the winds of change
are beginning to blow through its halls. Instead of Pizer's (1999) "corridors of excommunication," in which dissenting or challenging voices
are whispered about and discouraged, psychoanalysis seems to be inviting into its corridors, and even into its inner sanctums, new, questioning, vibrant voices prepared to enlarge and enliven the discourse in
which analysts engage. This is liberating and creates hope for all analysts and psychodynamically oriented therapists. For those who write
or speak in public, acceptance of the new, different, or divergent encourages us to stretch our voices, to reach for previously unsounded
notes, to play with unfamiliar accents and tones. For others, whose
voices are heard primarily in the consultation room, in schools, clin-
ics, hospitals, or community organizations, these trends offer greater
freedom to think more broadly about treatment and community issues
without feeling somehow in conflict with one's identity as an analyst
or psychodynamically oriented therapist or supervisor.

The process of teaching someone to do psychoanalytic therapy is
enormously complex. For example, how does one teach a supervisee to
surrender to experience, to subject that experience to thinking and

understanding, and then to relinquish thinking and understanding if they stand in the way of the therapeutic moment? So much of what supervisees need to learn is difficult to make explicit in words, and they too often hear, "I cannot explain to you how to do this if you have not experienced it yourself." And so as supervisors we strive to supplement our technical advice, our theoretical conceptions of the patient and of technique, with a relationship, a medium that is also the message. We embed our teachings in our own way of "being" and "doing" within the supervision. We do not take the supervisory process for granted, or ignore it, but rather recognize it as the carrier of so much of what we want to teach. We endeavor to engage supervisees in an experience that transmits, unconscious to unconscious, what we can never communicate directly or in words.

It is our hope that the experience of reading this book has similarly allowed the reader to receive a level of communication that goes deeper than the limits of our explicitly symbolized content. We hope the themes that we have been elaborating here—a relational view of the history of supervision and issues of authority, regression, teaching and treating, parallel process, case conference, and organizations—which have sprung so fully from our personal experiences, have enriched the reader's understanding and experience of the supervisory process and of the organizational life in which it transpires. Embedded within the historical and cultural moment at which we write, we as co-authors have raised our co-created third voice to articulate a model of supervision that incorporates contemporary approaches to psychoanalytic thinking and treatment paradigms. It is our hope that after completing this book, the reader will continue to elaborate, shape, and diverge from our ideas about the supervisory relationship, and to develop further another unique yet co-constructed psychodynamic voice.

References

Abramowitz, S., and Abramowitz, C. (1976). Sex role psychodynamics in psychotherapy supervision. *American Journal of Psychotherapy*, 39(4), 583–592.

Abrams, S. (1993). Reflections on supervisory models. *News from COPE*, 9(1), 4–6.

Altfeld, D., and Bernard, H. (1997). An experiential group model for group psychotherapy supervision. In C. Watkins (Ed.), *Handbook of Psychotherapy Supervision* (pp. 398–399). New York: Wiley.

Altman, N., and Davies, J. M. (2000). Editorial. *Psychoanalytic Dialogues*, 10, 1–4.

Arlow, J. (1963). The supervisory situation. *Journal of the American Psychoanalytic Association*, 11, 576–594.

Arlow, J., and Brenner, C. (1964). *Psychoanalytic Concepts and the Structural Theory*. New York: International Universities Press.

Aron, L. (1996). *A Meeting of Minds*. Hillsdale, NJ: Analytic Press.

Aron, L., and Bushra, A. (1998). Mutual regression: Altered states in the psychoanalytic situation. *Journal of the American Psychoanalytic Association*, 46(2), 389–412.

Balint, M. (1948). On the psychoanalytic training system. *Journal of Psycho-Analysis*, 29, 163–173.

Balint, M. (1957). Method and technique in the teaching of medical psychology. *British Journal of Medical Psychology*, 27, 37–41.

Balint, M. (1968). *The Basic Fault*. London: Tavistock.

Bassin, D. (1996). Beyond the he and she: Toward the reconciliation of masculinity and femininity in the postoedipal female mind. *Journal of the American Psychoanalytic Association*, 44(Suppl.), 157–190.

Baudry, F. (1993). The personal dimension and management of the supervisory situation with a special note on the parallel process. *Psychoanalytic Quarterly*, 62(4), 588–614.

Beebe, B., and Lachman, F. (1988). The contribution of mother–infant mutual influence to the origins of self and object representations. *Psychoanalytic Psychology*, 5, 303–337.

Benjamin, J. (1995). *Like Subjects, Love Objects*. New Haven, CT: Yale University Press.

Berman, E. (1997). Psychoanalytic supervision as the crossroads of a relational matrix.

In M. H. Rock (Ed.), *Psychodynamic Supervision* (pp. 167–188). Northvale, NJ: Jason Aronson.

Billow, R., and Mendelsohn, R. (1987). The peer supervisory group for psychoanalytic therapists. *Group*, 1, 35–46.

Bion, W. (1959). Attacks on linking. *International Journal of Psycho-Analysis*, 40, 308–315.

Bion, W. (1961). *Experiences in Groups*. London: Tavistock.

Bion, W. (1962). A theory of thinking. In *Second Thoughts* (pp. 110–119). New York: Aronson, 1967.

Brabant, E., Falzeder, E., and Giampieri-Deutsch, P. (Eds.). (1993). *The Correspondence of Sigmund Freud and Sandor Ferenczi: Vol. 1. 1908–1914*. Cambridge, MA: Belknap Press of Harvard University Press.

Brenner, C. (1982). *The Mind in Conflict*. Madison, CT: International Universities Press.

Breuer, J., and Freud, S. (1893–1895). Studies on Hysteria. In *Standard Edition*, 2, 1–311.

Brightman, B. (1984–85). Narcissistic issues in the training experience of the psychotherapist. *International Journal of Psychoanalytic Psychotherapy*, 10, 293–317.

Bromberg, P. (1991). On knowing one's patient inside out: The aesthetics of unconscious communication. *Psychoanalytic Dialogues*, 1(4), 399–422.

Bromberg, P. (1996). Standing in the spaces: Multiplicity of self in the psychoanalytic relationship. *Contemporary Psychoanalysis*, 32, 509–535.

Bromberg, P. (1998). *Standing in the Spaces*. Hillsdale, NJ: Analytic Press.

Bruzzone, M., Casaula, E., Jimenez, J., and Jordan, J. (1985). Regression and persecution in analytic training: Reflections on experience. *International Review of Psycho-Analysis*, 12, 411–415.

Buechler, S. (1996). Supervision of the treatment of borderline patients. *Contemporary Psychoanalysis*, 32, 86–92.

Bush, F. (1995). *The Ego at the Center of Clinical Technique*. Northvale, NJ: Jason Aronson.

Butler, J. (1995). Melancholy gender—Refused identification. *Psychoanalytic Dialogues*, 5(2), 165–180.

Caligor, L. (1984). Parallel and reciprocal processes in psychoanalytic supervision. In L. Caligor, P. Bromberg, and J. Meltzer (Eds.), *Clinical Perspective on the Supervision of Psychoanalysis and Psychotherapy* (pp. 1–28). New York: Plenum Press.

Caligor, L., Bromberg, P., and Meltzer, J. (Eds.). (1984). *Clinical Perspective on the Supervision of Psychoanalysis and Psychotherapy*. New York: Plenum Press.

Chodorow, N. (1992). Heterosexuality as a compromise formation: Reflections on the psychoanalytic theory of sexual development. *Psychoanalysis and Contemporary Thought*, 15(3), 267–304.

Christiansen, A. (1996). Masculinity and its vicissitudes: Reflections on some gaps in the psychoanalytic theory of male identity formation. *Psychoanalytic Review*, 83, 97–124.

Cooper, L., and Gustafson, J. (1985). Supervision in a group: An application of group theory. *The Clinical Supervisor*, 3(2), 7–25.

Courtois, C. A. (1988). *Healing the Incest Wound*. New York: Norton.

Crastnopol, M. (1999). The analyst's professional self as a "third" influence on the dyad. *Psychoanalytic Dialogues*, 9(4), 445–470.

Davies, J. M. (1994). Love in the afternoon: A relational reconsideration of desire and dread in the countertransference. *Psychoanalytic Dialogues*, 4, 153–170.

Davies, J. M. (1996). Linking the "pre-analytic" with the postclassical: Integration, dissociation, and the multiplicity of unconscious process. *Contemporary Psychoanalysis*, 32, 553–576.

Davies, J., and Frawley, M. (1994). *Treating the Adult Survivor of Childhood Sexual Abuse: A Psychoanalytic Perspective*. New York: Basic Books.

DeBell, D. (1981). Supervisory styles and positions. In R. Wallerstein (Ed.), *Becoming a Psychoanalyst* (pp. 39–60). New York: International Universities Press.

Dewald, P. (1987). *Learning Process in Psychoanalytic Supervision: Complexities and Challenges*. Madison, CT: International Universities Press.

Dimen, M. (1991). Deconstructing difference: Gender, splitting, and transitional space. *Psychoanalytic Dialogues*, 1(3), 335–352.

Doehrman, M. (1976). Parallel processes in supervision and psychotherapy. *Bulletin of the Menninger Clinic*, 40, 9–104.

Dupont, J. (Ed.). (1988). *The Clinical Diary of Sandor Ferenczi*. Cambridge, MA: Harvard University Press.

Dupont, J. (1993). Michael Balint: Analysand, pupil, friend, and successor to Sandor Ferenczi. In L. Aron and A. Harris (Eds.), *The Legacy of Sandor Ferenzci* (pp. 145–158). Hillsdale, NJ: Analytic Press.

Eckler-Hart, A. (1987). True and false self in the development of the psychotherapist. *Psychotherapy*, 24(4), 683–692.

Eissler, K. (1953). The effect of the structure of the ego on psychoanalytic technique. *Journal of the American Psychoanalytic Association*, 1, 104–143.

Ekstein, R., and Wallerstein, R. (1972). *The Teaching and Learning of Psychotherapy* (2nd ed.). New York: International Universities Press.

Eliot, T. S. (1942). Little gidding. In *Four Quartets* (p. 24). New York: Harcourt Brace.

Elise, D. (1998). Gender repertoire: Body, mind, and bisexuality. *Psychoanalytic Dialogues*, 8(3), 379–397.

Epstein, L. (1997). Collusive selective inattention to the negative impact of the supervisory situation. In M. Rock (Ed.), *Psychodynamic Supervision* (pp. 285–314). Northvale, NJ: Jason Aronson.

Erikson, E. (1963). *Childhood and Society*. New York: Norton.

Etchegoyen, R. H. (1991). *The Fundamentals of Psychoanalytic Technique*. London: Karnac.

Fairbairn, W. R. D. (1943). The repression and return of bad objects. In *Psychoanalytic Studies of the Personality* (pp. 59–81). London: Tavistock/Routledge, 1990.

Fairbairn, W. R. D. (1944). Endopsychic structure considered in terms of object relations. In *Psychoanalytic Studies of the Personality* (pp. 82–136). London: Tavistock/Routledge, 1990.

Fenichel, O. (1941). *Problems of Psychoanalytic Technique*. New York: Psychoanalytic Quarterly Press.

Ferenczi, S. (1932). Confusion of tongues between adults and the child. *International Journal of Psycho-Analysis*, 30, 225–229.

Fiscalini, J. (1997). On supervisory parataxis and dialogue. In M. H. Rock (Ed.), *Psychodynamic Supervision* (pp. 29–58). Northvale, NJ: Jason Aronson.

Fleming, J., and Benedek, T. (1966). *Psychoanalytic Supervision*. New York: Grune and Stratton.

Fortune, C. (1993). The case of "RN": Sandor Ferenczi's radical experiment in psychoanalysis. In L. Aron and A. Harris (Eds.), *The Legacy of Sandor Ferenczi* (pp. 101–120). Hillsdale, NJ: Analytic Press.

Fosshage, J. L. (1997). Towards a model of psychoanalytic supervision from a self-psychological/intersubjective perspective. In M. H. Rock (Ed.), *Psychodynamic Supervision* (pp. 189–212). Northvale, NJ: Jason Aronson.

Frawley-O'Dea, M. G. (1997a). Supervision amidst abuse: The supervisee's perspective. In M. H. Rock (Ed.), *Psychodynamic Supervision* (pp. 312–335). Northvale, NJ: Jason Aronson.

Frawley-O'Dea, M. G. (1997b). Who's doing what to whom? Supervision and sexual abuse. *Contemporary Psychoanalysis, 33*(1), 5–18.

Frawley-O'Dea, M. G. (1997c, February). *Supervision in the second century: A relational model of supervision*. Paper presented at the 17th annual spring meeting of the Division of Psychoanalysis (39) of the American Psychological Association, Denver, CO.

Frawley-O'Dea, M. G. (1998). Revisiting the "teach/treat" boundary in psychoanalytic supervision: When the supervisee is or is not in concurrent treatment. *Journal of the American Academy of Psychoanalysis, 26*, 513–528.

Freud, S. (1893). On the psychical mechanism of hysterical phenomena. *Standard Edition, 3*, 25–39.

Freud, S. (1900). The Interpretations of Dreams. *Standard Edition, 5*, 339–621.

Frijling-Schreuder, E. C. M. (1970). On individual supervision. *International Journal of Psycho-Analysis, 51*, 363–370.

Gabbard, G. O. (1999). Boundary violations and the psychoanalytic training system. *Journal of Applied Psychoanalytic Studies, 1*, 207–221.

Gabbard, G. O., and Lester, E. P. (1995). *Boundaries and Boundary Violations in Psychoanalysis*. New York: Basic Books.

Gardner, R. (1993). Reflections on the study group experience and on supervising. *News from COPE, 9*(1), 6–7.

Gay, P. (1988). *Freud*. New York: Doubleday.

Gediman, H., and Wolkenfeld, F. (1980). The parallelism phenomenon in psychoanalysis and supervision: Its reconsideration as a triadic system. *Psychoanalytic Quarterly, 49*, 234–255.

Gerson, S. (1996). Neutrality, resistance, and self-disclosure in an intersubjective psychoanalysis. *Psychoanalytic Dialogues, 6*(5), 623–645.

Goldner, V. (1991). Toward a critical relational theory of gender. *Psychoanalytic Dialogues, 1*(3), 249–272.

Gordon, R. (1995). The symbolic nature of the supervisory relationship: Identification and professional growth. *Issues in Psychoanalytic Psychology, 17*(2), 154–162.

Gray, P. (1990). The nature of the therapeutic action in psychoanalysis. *Journal of the American Psychoanalytic Association, 38*, 1083–1097.

Gray, P. (1994). *The Ego and Analysis of Defense*. Northvale, NJ: Jason Aronson.

Greenberg, J. (1995a). Psychoanalytic technique and the interactive matrix. *Psychoanalytic Quarterly, 64*, 1–22.

Greenberg, J. (1995b). Self-disclosure: Is it psychoanalytic? *Contemporary Psychoanalysis, 31*, 193–205.

Greenberg, J. (1996). Psychoanalytic words and psychoanalytic acts: A brief history. *Contemporary Psychoanalysis, 32*, 195–213.

Greenberg, J. (1999). Analytic authority and analytic restraint. *Contemporary Psychoanalysis, 35*(1), 25–41.

Grey, A., and Fiscalini, J. (1987). Parallel process as transference–countertransference interaction. *Psychoanalytic Psychology, 4*, 131–144.

Grinberg, L., Sor, D., and de Bianchedi, E. (1977). *Introduction to the Work of Bion*. New York: Jason Aronson.

Grotstein, J. S. (1985). *Splitting and Projective Identification*. Northvale, NJ: Jason Aronson.

Haber, R. (1996). *Dimensions of Psychotherapy Supervision*. New York: Norton.

Haesler, L. (1993). Adequate distance in the relationship between supervisor and supervisee: The position of the supervisor between "teacher" and "analyst." *International Journal of Psycho-Analysis, 74*(3), 547–555.

Harris, A. (1991). Symposium on Gender: Introduction. *Psychoanalytic Dialogues, 1*(3), 243–248.

Harris, A. (1996). The conceptual power of multiplicity. *Contemporary Psychoanalysis, 32*, 537–552.

Harris, A., and Ragen, T. (1995). Mutual supervision, countertransference, and self-analysis. In J. W. Barron (Ed.), *Critical Inquiries, Personal Visions* (pp. 196–216). Hillsdale, NJ: Analytic Press.

Hawes, S. (1992, January). *Reflexivity and Collaboration in the Supervisory Process: A Role for Feminist Poststructural Theories in the Training of Professional Psychologists*. Paper presented at the National Council of Schools of Professional Psychology Midwinter Conference on Clinical Training in Professional Psychology, Las Vegas, NV.

Herman, J. L. (1992). *Trauma and Recovery*. New York: Basic Books.

Hilpert, H. (1995). The place of the training group analyst and the problem of personal group analysis in block training. *Group Analysis, 28*, 301–311.

Hirsch, I. (1997). Supervision amidst abuse: The supervisor's perspective. In M. H. Rock (Ed.), *Psychodynamic Supervision* (pp. 339–360). Northvale, NJ: Jason Aronson.

Hirsch, I. (1998). Discussion of Frawley-O'Dea and Sarnat: Emotional and interactional factors in the supervisory relationship. *Journal of the American Academy of Psychoanalysis, 26*(4), 545–552.

Hoffman, I. Z. (1983). The patient as interpreter of the analyst's experience. *Contemporary Psychoanalysis, 19*, 389–422.

Hoffman, I. Z. (1991). Discussion: Toward a social-constructivist view of the psychoanalytic situation. *Psychoanalytic Dialogues, 1*, 74–105.

Hoffman, I. Z. (1992). Some practical implications of a social-constructivist view of the analytic situation. *Psychoanalytic Dialogues, 2*, 287–304.

Hoffman, I. Z. (1996). The intimate and ironic authority of the psychoanalyst's presence. *Psychoanalytic Quarterly, 63*(1), 187–218.

Hoffman, I. Z. (1998). *Ritual and Spontaneity in the Psychoanalytic Process*. Hillsdale, NJ: Analytic Press.

Holloway, E., and Wolleat, P. (1994). Supervision: The pragmatics of empowerment. *Journal of Educational and Psychological Consultation 5*(1), 23–43.

Horner, A. J. (1988). Developmental aspects of psychodynamic supervision: Parallel process of separation and individuation. *The Clinical Supervisor*, 6, 3–11.

Isakower, O. (1957). The analyzing instrument in the teaching and conduct of the analytic process. *Journal of Clinical Psychoanalysis*, 1, 181–194.

Issacharoff, A. (1984). Countertransference in supervision: Therapeutic consequences for the supervisee. In L. Caligor, P. M. Bromberg, and J. D. Meltzer (Eds.), *Clinical Perspectives on the Supervision of Psychoanalysis and Psychotherapy* (pp. 89–106). New York: Plenum Press.

Jacobs, D., David, P., and Meyer, D. (1995). *The Supervisory Encounter*. New Haven, CT: Yale University Press.

Janet, P. (1889). *L'automatisme psychologique*. Paris: Alcan.

Jarmon, H. (1990). The supervisory experience: An object relations perspective. *Psychotherapy*, 22(2), 195–201.

Jones, E. (1961). *The Life and Works of Sigmund Freud*. New York: Basic Books.

Josephs, L. (1990). The concrete attitude and the supervision of beginning psychotherapists. *Psychoanalysis and Psychotherapy*, 8(1), 11–22.

Kernberg, O. (1976). *Object Relations Theory and Clinical Psychoanalysis*. Northvale, NJ: Jason Aronson.

Kernberg, O. (1984). *Severe Personality Disorders*. New Haven, CT: Yale University Press.

Kernberg, O. (2000). A concerned critique of psychoanalytic education. *International Journal of Psycho-Analysis*, 81, 97–120.

Klein, M. (1946). Notes on some schizoid mechanisms. In *Envy and Gratitude and Other Works, 1946–1963* (pp. 282–311). New York: Delacorte, 1975.

Kluft, R. (1990). Incest and subsequent revictimization: The case of therapist–patient sexual exploitation, with a description of the sitting duck syndrome. In R. Kluft (Ed.), *Incest Related Syndromes of Adult Psychopathology* (pp. 263–288). Washington, DC: American Psychiatric Press.

Kohut, H. (1971). *The Analysis of the Self*. New York: International Universities Press.

Kohut, H. (1977). *The Restoration of the Self*. New York: International Universities Press.

Lacan, J. (1953). The function and field of speech and language in psycho-analysis. In *Ecrits: A Selection* (A. Sheridan, Trans., pp. 30–113). New York: Norton, 1977.

Lane, R. (Ed.). (1990) *Psychoanalytic Approaches to Supervision*. New York: Brunner/Mazel.

Langs, R. (1979). *The Supervisory Experience*. New York: Jason Aronson.

Langs, R. (1984). Supervisory crises and dreams from supervisees. In L. Caligor, P. Bromberg, and J. Meltzer (Eds.), *Clinical Perspectives on the Supervision of Psychoanalysis and Psychotherapy* (pp. 107–141). New York: Plenum Press.

Langs, R. (1994). *Doing Supervision and Being Supervised*. London: Karnac.

Lawner, P. (1989). Counteridentification, therapeutic impasse, and supervisory process. *Contemporary Psychoanalysis*, 25, 592–603.

Leary, K. (1997, February). *Supervision and Contemporary Clinical Practice: Deconstructing and Re-negotiating Clinical Authority in the Psychological Training Clinic*. Paper presented at the 17th Annual Spring Meeting of the Division of Psychoanalysis (39) of the American Psychological Association, Denver, CO.

Lebovici, S. (1970). Technical remarks on the supervision of psychoanalytic treatment. *International Journal of Psycho-Analysis, 51*, 385–392.

Leighton, J. (1991). Gender stereotyping in supervisory styles. *Psychoanalytic Review, 78*(3), 347–363.

Lesser, R. (1984). Supervision, illusions anxieties, and questions. In L. Caligor, P. Bromberg, and J. Meltzer (Eds.), *Clinical Perspectives on the Supervision of Psychoanalysis and Psychotherapy* (pp. 143–152). New York: Plenum Press.

Lester, E. P., and Robertson, B. M. (1995). Multiple interactive processes and psychoanalytic supervision. *Psychoanalytic Inquiry, 15*, 190–210.

Levenson, E. (1984). Follow the fox. In L. Caligor, P. Bromberg, and J. Meltzer (Eds.), *Clinical Perspectives on the Supervision of Psychoanalysis and Psychotherapy* (pp. 153–167). New York: Plenum Press.

Marshall, R. J. (1993). Perspectives on supervision: Tea and/or supervision? *Modern Psychoanalysis, 18*, 45–57.

Marshall, R. J. (1997). The interactional triad in supervision. In M. H. Rock (Ed.), *Psychodynamic Supervision* (pp. 77–106). Northvale, NJ: Jason Aronson.

May, R. (1986). Concerning a psychoanalytic view of maleness. *Psycho-Analytic Review, 73*, 175–193.

Meltzer, P. (1992). *The Claustrum*. Perthshire: Clunie Press.

Mendell, D. (1986). Cross-gender supervision of cross-gender therapy: Female supervisor, male candidate, female patient. *American Journal of Psychoanalysis, 46*(3), 270–275.

Mendell, D. (1993). Supervising female therapists: A comparison of dynamics while treating male and female patients. *Psychoanalytic Inquiry, 13*(2), 270–285.

Miller, L., and Twomey, J. E. (1999). A parallel without a process: A relational view of a supervisory experience. *Contemporary Psychoanalysis, 35*, 557–580.

Mitchell, S. A. (1988). *Relational Concepts in Psychoanalysis: An Integration*. Cambridge, MA: Harvard University Press.

Mitchell, S. A. (1993). *Hope and Dread in Psychoanalysis*. New York: Basic Books.

Mitchell, S. A. (1997). *Influence and Autonomy in Psychoanalysis*. Hillsdale, NJ: Analytic Press.

Mitchell, S. A., and Aron, L. (Eds.). (1999). *Relational Psychoanalysis*. Hillsdale, NJ: Analytic Press.

Mitchell, S., and Black, M. (1995). *Freud and Beyond*. New York: Basic Books.

Mordecai, E. (1991). A classification of empathic failures for psychotherapists and supervisors. *Psychoanalytic Psychology, 8*(3), 251–262.

Muller, J. (1999). The third as holding the dyad. *Psychoanalytic Dialogues, 9*(4), 471–480.

Nelson, M., and Holloway, E. (1990). Relation of gender to power and involvement in supervision. *Journal of Counseling Psychology, 37*, 473–481.

Newirth, J. (1990). The mastery of countertransferential anxiety: An object relations view of the supervisory process. In R. Lane (Ed.), *Psychodynamic Approaches to Supervision* (pp. 157–164). New York: Brunner/Mazel.

Ogden, T. (1982). *Projective Identification and Psychotherapeutic Technique*. Northvale, NJ: Jason Aronson.

Ogden, T. (1986). *The Matrix of the Mind*. Northvale, NJ: Jason Aronson.

Ogden, T. (1994). *Subjects of Analysis*. Northvale, NJ: Jason Aronson.

Ogden, T. (1997). *Reverie and Interpretation*. Northvale, NJ: Jason Aronson.

Panskepp, J. (1999). Emotions as viewed by psychoanalysis and neuroscience: An exercise in consilience. *Neuro-Psychoanalysis, 1*, 15–37.

Pegeron, J. (1996). Supervision as an analytic experience. *Psychoanalytic Quarterly, 65*(4), 693–710.

Pfeffer, D., Epstein, C., and Herrara, I. (1989). Group supervision: A psychodynamic perspective. In K. G. Lewis (Ed.), *Variations on Teaching and Supervising Group Therapy* (pp. 7–26). New York: Haworth Press.

Philipson, I. J. (1993). *On the Shoulders of Women: The Feminization of Psychotherapy*. New York: Guilford Press.

Pizer, B. (2000). Negotiating analytic holding: Discussion of Patrick Casement's *Leaning from the Patient. Psychoanalytic Inquiry, 20*(1), 82–107.

Pizer, S. (1996). The distributed self: Introduction to symposium on "The multiplicty of self and analytic technique." *Contemporary Psychoanalysis, 32*, 499–507.

Pizer, S. (1998). *Building Bridges: The Negotiation of Paradox in Psychoanalysis*. Hillsdale, NJ: Analytic Press.

Pizer, S. (1999, September). *Discussion of Paper by Joan Wheelis*. Paper presented at the Institute for Contemporary Psychoanalysis conference on psychoanalytic supervision, New York, NY.

Racker, H. (1957). The meanings and uses of countertransference. *Psychoanalytic Quarterly, 26*, 303–357.

Racker, H. (1968). *Transference and Countertransference*. Madison, CT: International Universities Press.

Rangell, L. (1968). The psychoanalytic process. *International Journal of Psycho-Analysis, 49*, 19–26.

Rangell, L. (1981). From insight to change. *Journal of the American Psychoanalytic Association, 29*, 119–141.

Reams, R. (1994). Selfobject transferences in supervision. *The Clinical Supervisor, 12*(2), 57–73.

Renik, O. (1995). The ideal of the anonymous analyst and the problem of self-disclosure. *Psychoanalytic Quarterly, 64*(3), 466–495.

Renik, O. (1999). Playing one's cards face up in analysis: An approach to the problem of self-disclosure. *Psychoanalytic Quarterly, 68*, 521–540.

Rioch, M. (1970). Group relations: Rationale and technique. *International Journal of Group Psychotherapy, 29*, 340–355.

Robertson, B., and Yack, M. (1993). A candidate dreams of her patient: A report and some observations on the supervisory process. *International Journal of Psycho-Analysis, 74*(5), 993–1003.

Rock, M. H. (Ed.). (1997). *Psychodynamic Supervision*. Northvale, NJ: Jason Aronson.

Rosbrow, T. (1997). From parallel process to developmental process: A developmental/plan formulation approach to supervision. In M. H. Rock (Ed.), *Psychodynamic Supervision* (pp. 213–236). Northvale, NJ: Jason Aronson.

Rosiello, F. W. (1989). Affective elements in supervision and parallel process. *Contemporary Psychotherapy Review, 5,* 54–70.

Sachs, D. M., and Shapiro, S. H. (1976). On parallel process in therapy and teaching. *Psychoanalytic Quarterly, 45,* 394–415.

Sarnat, J. (1992). Supervision in relationship: Resolving the teach–treat controversy in psychoanalytic supervision. *Psychoanalytic Psychology,* 9(3), 387–403.

Sarnat, J. (1997). The contribution of a process-oriented case conference to the development of students in the first year of a doctor of psychology training program. *The Clinical Supervisor,* 15(2), 163–180.

Sarnat, J. (1998). Rethinking the role of regressive experience in psychoanalytic supervision. *Journal of the American Academy of Psychoanalysis,* 26(4), 529–544.

Sarnat, R. (1952). Supervision of the experienced student. *Social Casework,* 33(4), 147–152.

Schecter, R. (1995). Supervisory transference. *Issues in Psychoanalytic Psychology,* 17(2), 163–168.

Schindelheim, J. (1995). Learning to learn, learning to teach. *Psychoanalytic Inquiry, 15,* 153–168.

Searles, H. S. (1955). The informational value of the supervisor's emotional experiences. *Psychiatry, 18,* 135–146.

Searles, H. S. (1962). Problems of psychoanalytic supervision. In *Collected Papers on Schizophrenia and Related Subjects* (pp. 584–604). New York: International Universities Press.

Seashore, C. (1975). *In Grave Danger of Growing: Observations on the Process of Professional Development.* Unpublished manuscript.

Singer, D. (1982). Professional socialization and adult development in graduate professional education. In B. Morrison (Ed.), *New Directions for Experiential Learning: Building on Experiences in Adult Development* (pp. 45–62). San Francisco: Jossey-Bass.

Skolnick, N. J., and Warshaw, S. C. (Eds.). (1992). *Relational Perspectives in Psychoanalysis.* Hillsdale, NJ: Analytic Press.

Slavin, J. (1997). Models of learning and psychoanalytic traditions. *Psychoanalytic Dialogues,* 7(6), 803–817.

Slavin, J. (1998). Influence and vulnerability in psychoanalytic supervision and treatment. *Psychoanalytic Psychology,* 15(2), 230–244.

Sloane, J. (1986). The empathic vantage point in supervision. In A. Goldberg (Ed.), *Progress in Self Psychology* (Vol. 2, pp. 188–211). New York: Guilford Press.

Slochower, J. (1996). *Holding and Psychoanalysis.* Hillsdale, NJ: Analytic Press.

Solnit, A. (1970). Learning from psychoanalytic supervision. *International Journal of Psycho-Analysis,* 51(3), 359–362.

Spezzano, C. (1993). *Affect in Psychoanalysis: A Clinical Synthesis.* Hillsdale, NJ: Analytic Press.

Spezzano, C. (1998). The triangle of clinical judgment. *Journal of the American Psychoanalytic Association,* 46(2), 365–388.

Steadman, J., and Harper, K. (1995). Group supervision of group psychotherapy. *Canadian Journal of Psychiatry, 40,* 484–488.

Stern, Daniel. (1985). *The Interpersonal World of the Infant.* New York: Basic Books.

Stern, Donnel. (1997). *Unformulated Experience.* Hillsdale, NJ: Analytic Press.

Stewart, H. (1992). *Psychic Experience and the Problems of Technique*. New York: Routledge.

Stimmel, B. (1995). Resistance to awareness of the supervisor's transferences with special reference to the parallel process. *International Journal of Psycho-Analysis, 76*, 609–618.

Stolorow, R. D., Orange, D. M., and Atwood, G. E. (1998). Projective identification begone! Commentary on paper by Susan H. Sands. *Psychoanalytic Dialogues, 8*, 719–726.

Strean, H. S. (1991). Colliding illusions among analytic candidates, their supervisors, and their patients: A major factor in some treatment impasses. *Psychoanalytic Psychology, 8*, 402–414.

Sullivan, H. S. (1956). *Clinical Studies in Psychology*. New York: Norton.

Tansey, M. J., and Burke, W. F. (1989). *Understanding Counter-Transference*. Hillsdale, NJ: Analytic Press.

Teitelbaum, S. (1990). Supertransference: The role of the supervisor's blind spots. *Psychoanalytic Psychology, 7*(2), 243–258.

Wagner, F. (1957). Supervision of psychotherapy. *American Journal of Psychotherapy, 11*, 759–768.

Wallerstein, R. (1981). *Becoming a Psychoanalyst*. New York: International Universities Press.

Weiss, J. (1993). *How Psychotherapy Works: Process and Technique*. New York: Guilford Press.

Wheelis, J. (1999, September). *Supervision as an Intersubjective Process*. Paper presented at the Institute for Contemporary Psychoanalysis conference on psychoanalytic supervision, New York, NY.

Winnicott, D. (1947). Hate in the countertransference. In *Through Paediatics to Psychoanalysis* (pp. 229–242). New York: Basic Books, 1975.

Winnicott, D. (1954). Withdrawal and regression. In *Through Paediatics to Psychoanalysis* (pp. 255–261). New York: Basic Books, 1975.

Wolkenfeld, F. (1990). The parallel process phenomenon revisited: Some additional thoughts about the supervisory process. In R. Lane (Ed.), *Psychoanalytic Approaches to Supervision* (pp. 95–109). New York: Brunner/Mazel.

Index

Abrams, S., 25, 30
Abstinence, therapist's, 56
  in handling regression, 106
Affective functioning
  in case conference, 203, 218
  case conference leader's role, 209, 218
  neurobiology, 179–180
Altfeld, D., 202–203
Altman N., 228–229
Analyst–centered supervision, 27
Anxiety of supervisor, 104–105
  in case conference, 203
Anxiety-focused (object relations)
    model, 39–41
Apologies, in therapeutic setting, 76
Arlow, J., 14, 136, 170, 172
Aron, L., 14–15, 17–18, 22–23, 57–58,
    73, 75–76, 81, 100, 108–110
Asymmetrical parallel process, 190–196
Asymmetry
  in analytic relationship, 54, 55, 58,
    60
  in supervisory relationship, 80–88
    evaluative component of
      supervision and, 60, 89–90
Authority of supervisor
  in case conference, 208
  co-creation of, 81–82
  conceptions of, in typology of
    supervision, 26
  during course of supervisory
    relationship, 78–79

in patient-centered model, 30
and positive supervisory atmosphere,
    74
postmodern perspective on, 74–80
as process, 82
in a relational model, 41, 59–61
in supervisee-centered models, 33, 34,
    37–38, 39
and supervisor as representative of
    external perspective, 92–96
See also Power relations

B

Balint, M., 14, 18–23, 107, 202, 221,
    226, 228
Basic assumption groups, 204–207
Baudry, F., 20, 170, 172–173, 181
Benedek, T., 1
Bernard, H., 202–203
Billow, R., 203
Bion, W., 10, 174, 178, 204, 206–
    207
Brabant, E., 16
Brightman, B., 29, 38, 42, 79, 113
Bromberg, P., 1, 51, 53, 108
Bruzzone, M., 114
Bushra, A., 57, 108–109

C

Caligor, L., 1, 122, 170, 172
Casaula, E., 114

241

Power relations
    in classical psychoanalytic theory and
        practice, 14, 15, 20, 22
    and conceptions of supervisor's
        authority, 26, 30, 33, 105
    evaluative component of supervision
        and, 89–90
    gender issues and, 99–103
    historical context of psychoanalytic
        theory and, 7, 13
    imbalance leading to relationship
        rupture and, 93–96
    negotiation in supervisory
        relationship and, 76
    organizational contexts and, 10–11
    recognition of, 83–84
    regressive response to supervisor and,
        113–116
    relational model of supervision, 8,
        59–61
    relational model of therapy, 57–58
    sexual boundaries in supervision and,
        97
    supervisor as representative of
        professional community and,
        92–93
    in therapeutic relationship, 8
Process-centered supervision, 27
Projective identification
    function of, 178
    neurobiology and, 179–180
    in parallel process, 175–179
    psychoanalytic conceptualizations of,
        174–175
    relational theory and, 178
    therapeutic approach and, 178
Psychoanalytic theory and practice, 2
    classical theory, 14–15, 16, 28, 106
    current models of supervision and,
        25, 28–42
    current trends in supervision and,
        23–24
    eclectic practice and, 42
    historical evolution of, 7, 13, 197
    historical models of supervision and,
        15, 16–22, 28–33

practice as craft and, 60–61
    range of approaches in, 7–8, 20
    regression in, 8–9, 106–107
Psychopathology, relational theory of,
    52–53

R

Ragen, T., 20, 137, 154, 167
Regression
    analyst's, 57
    case transcript illustration, 124–135
    conservative approach, 109–112
    definition and characteristics, 107–
        109
    inevitability of, 108
    mutual regulation of, 120
    psychoanalytic theory and, 8–9, 106–
        107
    range of experiences and, 107
    relational approach to, 56–57
    in relational model of supervision,
        65–69
    as response to learning, 116–122
    significance of, in supervision, 9, 106,
        107, 108, 109, 135
    sources of, 112
    and supervisee response to patient,
        113
    and supervisee response to supervisor,
        113–116
    in supervisor, 122–124
    supervisory focus on, 110–112
    therapeutic significance of, 108–109
Relational theory and practice
    and analyst's authority, 57–58, 59–61
    and case conference model, 201,
        207–218
    clinical features of, 2–3, 69–70
    and concept of psychopathology, 52–
        53
    and concept of self, 51–52
    conceptual basis of, 50–58
    and construction of meaning in
        therapy, 54–55
    didactic aspect of supervision in, 31